MIRRORS OF MADNESS

Patrolling the Psychic Border

SOCIAL PROBLEMS AND SOCIAL ISSUES

An Aldine de Gruyter Series of Texts and Monographs

SERIES EDITORS

John I. Kitsuse, *University of California, Santa Cruz*
Joseph W. Schneider, *Drake University*

Images of Issues: Typifying Contemporary Social Problems
Joel Best (Editor)

Constructing Social Problems
Malcolm Spector and John I. Kitsuse

Mirrors of Madness: Patrolling the Psychic Border
Bruce Luske

MIRRORS OF MADNESS

Patrolling the Psychic Border

Bruce Luske

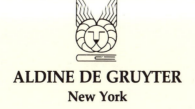

ALDINE DE GRUYTER
New York

ABOUT THE AUTHOR

Bruce Luske is Professor of Sociology in the Graduate School of Education and Human Development at the University of Rochester, New York. He received his B.A. at Sonoma State University and his Ph.D. at the University of California, Santa Cruz. His many interests include social problems, critical theory, postmodernism, and popular culture.

ALDINE DE GRUYTER
A Division of Walter de Gruyter, Inc.
200 Saw Mill River Road
Hawthorne, New York 10532

Library of Congress Cataloging-in-Publication Data

Luske, Bruce, 1944-
    Mirrors of madness:patrolling the psychic border/Bruce Luske.
        p.   cm. — (Social problems and social issues)
    Includes bibliographical references.
    Includes index.
    ISBN 0-202-30422-1. — ISBN 0-202-30423-X(pbk.)
    1. Mental health personnel and patient.   2. Mental health
personnel—Mental health.   3. Social psychiatry.   I. Title.
II. Series.
RC480.8.L87   1990
616.89'023—dc20   90-37210
                                                                             CIP

Printed in the United States of America

10 9 8 7 6 5 4 3 2 1

We can get to the age of understanding and wisdom, and the power behind that is the power of love, which will conquer the love of power.

Kate, labeled psychotic

CONTENTS

PREFACE

This book has had a very long period of development. In fact, it started to form when I began doing psychiatric work in the 1970s. From the beginning I noticed that the jargon used in this work had a powerful influence on the personal realities of all involved with it. And I had this insight long before I believed, having become a sociologist in 1986, that the words we use do indeed constitute reality for us. I hope, of course, that my portrayal of psychiatric realities here will make some small contribution toward persuading colleagues, as yet unconvinced of this premise, that "social constructionism" is not just another competing sociological paradigm but, frankly, all there is.

This book is written not only (or even primarily) for sociologists, psychologists, or other "social service professionals," but also for curious and literate students and lay people. I have tried to make it accessible to the ordinary person. Most of all, it is written for those having direct experience of the psychiatric enterprise. Which is not to say that readers will necessarily *like* or *agree* with my construction of this psychiatric world. To paraphrase the late sociologist C. Wright Mills, I have tried to be fair but am never neutral. I make no apology for the fact that this study is inspired by advocacy for the recipients of psychiatric intervention.

So considered, in 1983 I began the field study on which this book is based centering my attention mainly on the labeled-psychotic residents of a psychiatric halfway house. My exclusive goal at that time was to examine the sociological consequences of psychiatric care for those so designated. While the book retains this concern, the staff's application of psychiatric definitions not only to the situations of residents but to those of their own lives gradually emerged as the predominant theme. The book as a whole, then, is intended to show how psychiatric work creates patterns of interaction between the staff and residents that routinely poses the question, "Who's crazy?" on both the individual and societal levels. Thus, alongside the primary focus on the psychiatric setting, I also intend the book to embody an always implicit and sometimes explicit critique of the American social order.

Let me now very briefly introduce the chapters to follow. In Chapter 1, "Constructing Psychiatric Reality," I argue that social-constructionist methods ought to be wed to critical theory in studying social problems. I also focus this perspective on the ideology and organization of institutional psychiatry and its problematic relationship with capitalist institutions. Finally, after introducing the institutional context and organizational roles of the specific psychiatric setting, I discuss some concrete methodological issues involved in the study.

Chapter 2, "Border Crossing," shows how people pass into a labeled-psychotic status in this setting. Then residents so defined describe their families and social backgrounds. Next, the nature of psychiatric intervention into residents' lives in the setting, including the issue of psychiatric drugs, is described and analyzed in terms of how these practices influence their social status and personal identities.

In Chapter 3, "Border Patrol," staff families and social backgrounds, cultural orientations, and the relationships between these dimensions and avenues into psychiatric work are described and analyzed. The rest of the chapter is taken up with the depiction and analysis of staff devices for distinguishing themselves from the residents both socially and psychologically.

Chapter 4, "Border Lines," is concerned with comparative analysis of "unusual experiences" as defined and described by residents and staff. This chapter also extends the description and analysis (begun in the previous chapter) of staff strategies, imbedded in their work, which are intended to maintain the border between the staff's "sanity" and the residents' "insanity"—and ward off the special threat posed by the labeled-"borderline" residents.

In Chapter 5, "Border Disputes," direct skirmishes between staff and residents over the nature and location of the border between "sanity" and "insanity" are described and analyzed. Also, I examine the effects of these conflicts and the other burdens on veteran staff of patrolling the border.

The concluding chapter, "Borderland," reviews major points from the descriptions and analyses comparing residents and staff in the preceding four chapters, summarizes their basic social-psychological and institutional dimensions—my "map" of this psychiatric territory—and indicates some theoretical and methodological direction for future study suggested by these materials.

A final note before we begin: I believe that sociological work ought to aim at evoking a thoughtful reexamination of taken-for-granted personal and institutional practices. This is my primary goal in this work. And whether or not one succeeds in this objective often has nothing to do with popular appeal. Indeed, since this self-reflexive process is often person-ally painful, "success" in these terms can mean exactly the opposite. Whatever your response to the nature of my methods or analysis, I sincerely hope that you derive something of humane value and personal usefulness from the portrayals in these pages.

Bruce Luske

ACKNOWLEDGMENTS

This book has been influenced by many people. I want first to express my gratitude to the psychiatric staff and residents who let me into their lives. I did my honest best to express their sociological situations. And speaking of sociological situations, I would not be writing these acknowledgments (because there might not have been a book) were it not for the patient encouragement of the writing and wonderful personal support of my editors, John Kitsuse and Joseph Schneider. Further, their perceptive editorial suggestions have made this a better book than it might have been otherwise.

I also want to thank the following people: Harvey Segal, Kay Trimberger, Richard Appelbaum, Richard Lichtman, Peter Lyman, John Alexander, and Bev Bacak for being, in very different and crucial ways, important influences, "role models," and friends. I am especially thankful also for the close friendship of Hank Vandenburgh, whose brilliance through the years has greatly benefited this work; and for the insight and empathy of Jane Jordan and Cleo Barber, who have enabled me to prevail. And most prominently, I am deeply grateful to Sonja Saint Amant, whose loving support—not to mention sociological and literary talent and sharp editoral eye for weaknesses in my text—have greatly influenced whatever strengths I and the book may embody. My and its shortcomings, however, are entirely my responsibility. Finally, special thanks to Trev Leger and the other people at Aldine de Gruyter for their very helpful assistance and patience.

Chapter 1

CONSTRUCTING PSYCHIATRIC REALITY

Some guy scales a skyscraper in midtown Manhattan. At the edge of the same city, another guy parachutes into a ballpark during the World Series as 50,000 people at the game and millions more watching on TV look on in amazement. A man in Chicago snarls rush hour traffic by running onto State Street and proclaiming that he is the son of God. In Los Angeles, the "Hillside strangler" stalks women one by one. Whether repelled or riveted, we Americans have an insatiable hunger for tales of bums, winos, killers, "kooks," "commies," and "creeps"— "oddballs" of all types.

Why do we have this love/hate affair with the lunatic fringe? Is there too little room in our massively machined and computer disk–driven lives for adventure, drama, and reverie? Do we want "proof" that heros and villains, gods and devils, still exist? That, despite everything, extraordinary parts of ourselves can prevail?

In any case, we do act desperate for something—anything—to help us rise above the leveled landscape of daily routine. The following study of psychiatry draws on this need to peer past the outer limits of the ordinary to the extraordinary. But before "traveling" to the border of this strange land, we need to consider what conceptual tools we ought to "pack" to help us get by there.

Constructing Society: Theory

My background model for this study views social reality as "invention" and "construction." Invention means not only innovative thought or activity, but includes all human doings as inherently imaginative (Wagner 1981). Like Shakespeare's, this "dramaturgical" model (Goffman 1959:74) sees the social world as a vast stage, and people as actors.

1

Social life is produced as device and contrivance through processes of symbolic interaction. Sincerely or cynically, we present ourselves in the costumes and masks of our social roles *as* social reality (Nietzsche 1967). Society becomes drama and theater: art (Berger 1963).

The kindred constructionist standpoint (Berger and Luckmann 1967) likens the social world as a "house," which people build and maintain. If people find their inherited home too small, they can knock out a wall or add a room. If they require more light, larger windows can be installed. If the foundation is crumbling or the walls rotting with termites, the house can be renovated or razed. A new home can be "constructed" in its place. Or, people may decide that their abode is sound, only needs minor repairs or paint—and maybe new furniture and drapes.

Our lives are ongoing mutual creations. Like a jazz group, we improvise events through a combination of our histories and instruments. We question our pasts with imaginations stretched toward the future. But there is no end to *this* piece—in the final analysis, there is no "final analysis." The welter of events in their entirety escapes our grasp. We can only continue to express ourselves to each other from diverse vantage points in the hope that our "music" will be well received.

We tell one another stories about reality *as if* we know it. Our geniuses tell us stories, play music, paint pictures, which we find profound insofar as we see ourselves in them. Genius is that rare ability to stir us to the full throb of life in its limits and possibilities—its joys, passions, sorrows, and terrors. Few have written like Shakespeare or composed like Beethoven, but we lesser mortals, when immersed in their works, are empowered to touch our divinity, and so to divine the portentous truths and exquisite beauties that are life.

The invention and constructionist standpoints see people as architects of their existence. Though we live within material constraints—environmental, biological, and economic—we actively create and rearrange our social world.

This approach can make sense of any social setting, but it also holds that no interpretation of the social world is adequate to its structure. No human model (ironically, including this one) is capable of sustaining a metaphysical claim to reflect the world as it "really is." No court of appeal can render the final verdict on the nature of "objective reality." Truth is provisional and plural. This is human invention:

> The perspective I have developed here is not simply anomalous or divergent from our academic or secular ideologies, but directly contradictory of them. It suggests that the very realities upon which we base our theories, actions and institutions are contrivances of human invention and conventional interpretation. (Wagner 1981:157)

Thus my work exploring psychiatry is one sociologist's bridge to you, not a pipeline to reality. The latter approach would only create another lifeless sociological fossil. I hope, of course, that my eye is keen enough to sketch accounts that ring true to you. In any case, to paraphrase the marvelous old TV show, "The Naked City," "There are eight million stories in the naked city—this will be one of them."

Constructing Social Problems

The constructionist approach to social problems (Spector and Kitsuse 1987; Schneider and Kitsuse 1984) grew out of the "labeling theory" of deviance (Lemert 1951; Kitsuse 1962). The labeling standpoint emphasizes that social life is the ongoing creation of interacting individuals and groups. This perspective has been concerned mainly with interaction between alleged deviants and agencies of social control (e.g., police, legal, and medical authorities). It focuses on the latter groups because they are thought to wield greater power to determine what behavior is defined, and thus created, as deviant (Warren and Johnson 1970).[1]

The heir of labeling theory, the constructionist view focuses on the claims–making by different groups as to what constitutes a social problem. It expands the core idea of labeling theory that "deviant behavior is behavior that people so label" (Becker 1963:9) into the like idea that an activity becomes a "social problem" only if so defined. In fact, a social problem does not exist unless defined as such.

As in labeling theory, the likelihood of an activity becoming a social problem depends mainly on its public visibility and on the relative power of different groups to define it so. Its main thrust also proceeds from interactional to organizational levels of analysis. Finally, it too assumes that the character of agencies of social control—from family to government—results from the negotiation of these contending claims.

For example, suppose that an ecologist in 1940 claimed that the planet would die within 100 years unless productive and ecological practices in the West were radically altered. At that time few people supported this view of the "problem." Ecology was an obscure and specialized science. Certainly no social movement acted on this dire prediction. But today an international movement is working to save the environment—even as the planet lurches toward extinction.

An example from my study will serve to illustrate the constructionist view. Psychiatric staff often privately worry about their self-defined "odd" experiences. Especially if revealed within the psychiatric setting, experiences like those of the patients could be construed as symptoms of mental illness. But these ruminations do not become a *social* problem insofar as staff avoid revealing them publicly. Even were these experiences to leak into public view, staff have the social legitimacy, and therefore the power, to define them as "normal." Their charges, however, as the public exponents of the social problems known as "mental illness," are granted no legitimate power of definition.

The constructionist approach addresses the following questions:

1. How are the activities of some people defined as a social problem by others (including which group has greater power to impose its definition as "reality")?
2. What is the empirical content of the activity defined as a social problem?
3. What empirical processes construct the social problem?

The approach also views social problems as having a "career" or "natural history": They are seen as typically developing through four stages, briefly summarized as follows:

Stage 1: Group(s) attempt to assert the existence of some condition, define it as offensive, harmful, or otherwise undesirable, publicize these assertions, stimulate controversy, and create a public or political issue over the matter.

Stage 2: Recognition of the legitimacy of these group(s) by some official organization, agency, or institution. This may lead to an official investigation, proposals for reform, and the establishment of an agency to respond to those claims and demands.

Stage 3: Reemergence of claims and demands by the original group(s), or by others, expressing dissatisfaction with the established procedures for dealing with the imputed conditions, the bureaucratic handling of complaints, the failure to generate a condition of trust and confidence in the procedures, and the lack of sympathy for the complaints.

Stage 4: Rejection by complainant group(s) of the agency's or institution's response, or lack of response to their claims and demands, and the development of activities to create alternative, parallel, or counterinstitutions as responses to the established procedures (Spector and Kitsuse 1977:142).[2]

The analytic design of this framework expresses the view that "objectivity" (i.e., social policy on social problems) results from the interplay and contention of multiple group perspectives on the world. This pluralistic theory of knowledge harbors no exclusive moral or political commitments in its procedures. Accordingly, its empirical method simply intends to describe, without judgment, the full range of claims-making activities by groups constructing the social problem.

The constructionist standpoint holds that there can be no certainty about the truth of value orientations. But it also sees value commitments as inevitable, and moral neutrality as therefore impossible (Becker 1967). Thus this perspective ought not be construed as a totally relativistic, "anything goes" approach to the study of social life. On the contrary, well-reasoned moral and political stands on social issues are called for. And this point suggests the idea of a critical theory of social problems.

Critically Constructing Social Problems

The constructionist view stresses that people actively create social life. It also holds, however, that the nature of this creation mostly reflects which groups hold greater power to impose their definitions of social reality (including what constitutes a social problem) on others. In both respects it is highly compatible with the "critical theory" tradition of social thought (Jay 1973; Bernstein 1976; Held 1982; Watson 1982; Warren 1984).

Critical theory holds that people are world-makers who can search "beyond the details of social life to the conditions that shape existence. . . . [It] constantly reasons that no social arrangement is inevitable or beyond question" (Watson 1982:232). Its historic project is to de-reify the future by challenging the power of predefinition and the definitions of the powerful. Critical theory can be usefully crystallized as follows:

> Critical Sociology studies society as a totality and in its historical setting from the viewpoint of criticism and social-political practice, i.e., with a view not only to making visible what happens anyhow, but rather to making us aware of and keeping us aware of what we must *do;* viz. the planning and shaping of the future which we cannot avoid being engaged in. (G. Radnitsky in Watson 1982:231–232)[3]

Critical theory *(theoria)* inherently presupposes action *(praxis)* expressing its moral commitment to a freer world. It therefore seeks practical guides to action dismantling the domination it sees behind all historic constructions of society. The purpose of social inquiry is to critique what presently exists in terms of what it suppresses. The overarching task, then, is to cast doubt on all official versions of social reality and "what everybody knows" so as to spark insights into social arrangements in the interest of humane social change.

However, critical theory to date has been deeply flawed by its inability to ground itself in the practical interests of ordinary people. If not brought down to earth, its critique will always and deservedly evaporate into elite thin air. Accordingly, my chief purpose in introducing the constructionist approach to social problems here is that in my judgment it provides the most empirically insightful and practical framework for redressing this defect.

Psychiatry as a Social Problem

Institutional psychiatry currently is the only legitimate official agency for addressing ordinary people's "problems in living."[4] And psychiatric hegemony continues to grow through successful claims that all manner of individual psychic pain is evidence of "mental illness." (Conrad and Schneider 1980; Szasz 1984). Two recent sociological accounts of the statistical evidence of mental illness (though not the intent of the authors) illustrate the extent of this process:

> According to a recent study of the National Institute of Mental Health (NIMH), 19 percent of American adults suffer from at least one psychiatric disorder in any given period of 6 months, and 29–38 percent have been mentally ill at least once in their lifetime. . . . The NIMH study did not include the patients of mental hospitals and institutions. Nor did it include the homeless, many of whom suffer from mental disorder. In addition, 13 percent of the individuals originally chosen to be interviewed refused, and people in another 5–10 percent of the households refused to identify their relatives slated to be interviewed. (Thio 1988:303–304)

> The National Institute of Mental Health reported that in 1975 approximately 15 percent of Americans had some type of mental illness. Additionally, perhaps 80 percent of the populations have mild psychiatric symptoms at some point in their lives. . . . There were 1.7 million cases of treated mental disorder in 1955. By 1975, that figure rose to 6.4 million cases. These figures do not include . . . the 1 in 8 Americans that suffer serious depression at some point in their lives . . . [or] patients under the care of psychiatrists in private practice, clinical psychologists, various types of 'counselors,' or psychiatric social workers. (Gallagher 1987:2–3)

What do these statistics mean? At minimum they assume that mental illness is an objective and measurable social and psychological fact. Their magnitude also suggests a grave dislocation in the well-being of many people. But much sociological evidence also indicates that the psychiatric definitional claims (diagnoses) and clinical practices (treatment) behind the figures ironically create or worsen people's difficulties (cf. Nunally 1961; Goffman 1961, 1971; Phillips 1963; Scheff 1975; Temerlin 1968; Rosenhan 1973; Estroff 1981). The people in Thio's account who refused to be interviewed or to identify relatives as potentially mentally ill may have been onto something. Institutional psychiatry may constitute the greater social problem than the legions of people so defined under its sway.

Capitalism as the Social Problem

My critique of this "psychiatrization" of America contends that the bad fit between the social institutions of late capitalism and human desire and need produces this psychic pain, which psychiatry is increasingly called upon to contain. As critic David Ingleby puts it:

> Psychiatry . . . protects the efficient functioning of these institutions by converting the conflict and suffering that arises within them into 'symptoms' of essentially individual (or at best familial) 'malfunctioning.' It thus attempts to provide short-term technological solutions to what are at root policital problems. (Ingleby 1980:44)

However, this critical view of psychiatry and capitalism, like all other claims, has no privileged or exclusive ability to reflect the real world. It reflects a moral commitment to a particular vision and method for achieving a freer world. But since this perspective now has few advocates (cf. Ingleby 1980; Kovel 1980; O'Connor 1987), it must contend practically with opposing claims. Unless people have the desire *and* power to define and institutionalize an activity or situation as a social problem, no social problem exists "objectively." My hope, of course, is that this inquiry into psychiatry and the social order will be persuasive and telling enough to spur this support.

I have contended that the constructionist perspective offers great empirical insight and usefulness. My claim only wants to expand this perspective's traditional and crucial focus on the organization of agencies of social control to include that of world capitalism. In my view, the latter structure has emerged historically (cf. Polanyi 1944; Wallerstein 1978) as the central moral/political social force that most constrains and influences (not causes) the development of the social agencies and problems constructionists have addressed. I am convinced that the constructionist perspective can realize its potential only by joining its empirical imagination to the holistic insight of critical theory in the interest of human emancipation from all invidious and oppressive social divisions, most centrally those of class, gender, and race.

Psychiatric Ideology

In contrast to the constructionist and critical theory standpoints, psychiatry embraces a positivistic theory of knowledge. Positivism holds that scientific method is the *only* valid path of knowledge. It seeks objective knowledge—precisely definable, measurable, and based on lawful generalizations of cause and effect—in order to predict and control the physical and social world. The statistical overviews of "mental illness" by sociologists Thio and Gallagher presented above also refect this perspective.

Constructionists agree that science provides an important, indeed, profound way through which people make experience intelligible, morally viable, and useful. The productions of pioneering scientists and artists, for example, Einstein and Picasso, have great imaginative inventiveness in common. And scientific logic as expressed in technology forms the basis of physical survival upon which all other cultural creation depends (Habermas 1972).

However, constructionists reject the exclusivity of this faith, which calls all forms of knowledge departing from its canon of objective explanation irrational, and therefore false. This book itself is part of a series intended to contend with the positivism (mis)informing the dominant position in sociology. Constructionists find no bedrock of objective reality under the interpretations of people. Social "facts" reflect the value orientations of observers—including advocates of positivism (Kuhn 1970). In short, social objectivity is always the subjectivity of some group.

The psychiatric view of "mental illness" derives from the disease model of Western medicine, which has its historic roots in positivism (Manning and Zucker 1976). I shall only briefly outline aspects of this model, presented in great detail elsewhere (Shershow 1978), as an introduction to the psychiatric ideology of psychosis central to this study.

Emil Kraepelin (1904) is credited with developing the disease model for psychosis, which he called "dementia praecox." This analytic framework is still at the center of contemporary psychiatry (Shershow 1978):

1. A specific biological cause, i.e., defective brain structure or biochemical malfunction, underlies psychosis. Both maladies are thought to have genetic origins.
2. Psychosis has a characteristic developmental sequence, or stages.
3. These stages progress until the disease terminates in death (rarely), cure (rarely), or, most frequently, permanent disability.
4. The characteristics (symptoms) of psychosis are measurable and classifiable (diagnoses) by general and specific types—and are treatable by therapy.

The Swiss psychiatrist Eugene Bleuler (1924) is credited with coining the diagnosis "schizophrenia," which replaced the earlier "dementia praecox." He further elaborated its general symptoms and classified its specific types. The basic features that psychiatry still views as constituting schizophrenia are:

1. Social isolation and withdrawal are universal features.
2. Conceptual disorganization to the point of incomprehensibility is most often involved.
3. Profound emotional apathy and physical lethargy are almost always present.
4. Thought disorder or "delusions" are frequently present. (Delusions are uncorroborated beliefs in the reality of phenomena.)
5. Perceptual disorder or "hallucinations" are universal features. (Hallucinations are uncorroborated claims to hear or see phenomena.) The presence of hallucinations is the key indicator of schizophrenia, and auditory hallucinations are thought to occur far more often than visual hallucinations.

Community Psychiatry

My purpose here is not to provide a thorough account of the structure, history, and politics of the psychiatric industry (cf. Rothman 1971; Chu and Trotter 1974; Illich 1976, Scull 1977, 1981; Conrad and Schneider 1980; Ingleby 1980; Kovel 1980; Doerner 1984). I simply want to set the stage for my research and orient the reader by briefly sketching the institutional web that ensnares the cast of characters in the piece.

The organizational setting of this study is located within the community psychiatric system in California. The community psychiatric movement began in California during the mid-1960s. This movement was the result of an unusual coalition of then Governor Ronald Reagan, his conservative allies in the nursing home industry, and middle-class psychiatric professionals—especially social workers who were quite critical of the state hospitals (Vandenburgh 1979).[5] At that time the state mental hospitals were full of patients initially placed there by social agencies responding to doctors who proffered "somatic cures," e.g., electroshock and lobotomy, for mental problems. However, over time the huge increase in numbers of these so-called chronically mentally ill people suggested to critics that psychiatry's curative abilities were problematic. As large, visible eyesores, these asylums increasingly became the target of a "humanistic" crusade alleging that they merely "warehoused," neglected, and abused their charges. In fact, some reforms in the state hospitals—e.g., sharp reductions in somatic procedures—were achieved as a by-product of this movement.

During the 1960s, critics of psychiatry and social workers helped to generate a movement to reintegrate these patients into the community. Using such atypical examples as Gheel, Belgium—a traditional village that has succored the disordered for several centuries—they argued that the urban American community could provide the same forms of solidary support. In contrast, it was claimed, the asylum was a "total institution" where such support was wholly lacking. But the wholesale transfer during the 1960s and 1970s of large numbers of patients from the state hospitals to local communities did not result in the greater support for patients promised by these claims-makers. Instead, this successful construction of the asylum as social problem led to the subsequent, and virtually unchallenged, situation of patients crowded into slum boarding homes or convalescent hospitals, which served the same function as state hospitals but used cheaper labor (Vandenburgh 1979).

The chief beneficiaries of the community psychiatric movement have been psychiatric professionals and nursing home interests. The former group saw in this movement a way to challenge medical psychiatry's virtual monopoly over psychiatric policy, as well as the opportunity for increased influence on its direction. They failed in their first objective, but succeeded in obtaining more lucrative and influential jobs as middle managers and clinicians within the burgeoning psychiatric bureaucracies. And the nursing home industry as a whole has turned a tidy profit from the government transfers, i.e., taxes, from which state medical insurance pays for treatment in the community (Vandenburgh 1979).

The ironic result of this unlikely political alliance has been a far-flung, *geographically* decentralized psychiatric system that nonetheless remains under the exclusive control of the medical establishment. If anything, the medical grip on psychiatric policy has intensified. As for the patient population, or "clientele" most affected by this policy, there is largely an illusion of effective treatment as they are shuttled from stop to stop in the system.

There are six of these major stops in California's present psychiatric system:[6]

1.   Locked "acute" psychiatric hospitals, typically the point of entry into the system, house people viewed as a clear and present danger to themselves or others, or as presently unable to provide for their food, clothing, and shelter, i.e., as "gravely disabled."

2.   Unlocked "subacute" facilities also house people seen as gravely disabled, but who have stabilized enough psychologically to benefit from clinical treatment aimed at reintegrating them into normal society.

3.   Locked nursing homes, i.e., "skilled nursing" or long-term facilities, house people viewed as *chronically* gravely disabled or as a threat to themselves or others. Since rehabilitation of these people is regarded as most unlikely, clinical treatment consists primarily of custodial maintenance.

4.   Unlocked "board and care" facilities house people considered to be chronically disabled in the above sense, but who have stabilized enough to live quasi-independently in normal society. These facilities have no rehabilitative clinical component, but provide shelter, food, and minimal custodial supervision.

5.   Of course, the primarily locked state hospitals remain (and indications are that they are filling up again) for the "chronically disabled" who have exhausted the resources of facilities in local communities (often a coded expression to mean those who have exceeded the political tolerance of local agencies of social control).

6.   The final and perhaps chief stop since the advent of community psychiatry are slum hotels, other substandard housing, or the streets —homelessness. This stop is typical for the chronically disabled who are discharged or escape from psychiatric facilities, or otherwise fall through the cracks of the system. And the cracks loom large, indeed, when one considers that the subacute facility in East Lake County (stop 2, and the setting for this study) has 14 beds for a population of over 200,000 people.

The Organizational Setting

The site of this study is a community psychiatric facility in California. Its name and location—Eastside Psychiatric Intervention Center (EPIC) in East Lake county—however, are fictional. A useful way to see EPIC in terms of its manifest purpose is as a halfway house between the poles of mental hospitalization as a starting point and independent living in the community as the ideal clinical goal. EPIC is administered by Psychiatric Intervention Community Services (PICS), also a fictional name, which is its parent company. PICS is a nonprofit, tax-exempt private corporation under contract with East Lake County to provide subacute services for its residents. An extended excerpt from PICS' *Annual Report 1981–82* on the performance of EPIC follows:[7]

[The] EPIC [center in] Lakeside was opened in November, 1980 as an open, unlocked, voluntary 14-bed, short-term social rehabilitation program for acute mentally ill adults. During its second year of operation (1981–82) EPIC provided services to 103 clients with an average length of stay of approximately seven weeks. . . The typical EPIC client . . . was a relatively young (mean age: 27.5 years) person who had experienced approximately seven prior hospitalizations before coming to EPIC. . . 95% of clients . . . had prior admits to psychiatric hospitals and more than half (61%) had spent time in either state hospitals or long-term "L" facilities. A very high percentage (85%) of the 103 clients were diagnosed as psychotic with 74%

given a diagnosis of schizophrenia. Eighty-five of the 103 had resided previously in a board and care home or 24-hour residential program ["L" facility, state hospital—or EPIC itself]. Factors precipitating admission to EPIC indicate that a substantial percentage of clients (73%) were suffering from acute psychotic symptoms at intake with 10% evidencing suicidal symptoms. . . .

The typical EPIC client emerges as one who manifests a high level of mental and emotional disturbance with a significant previous history of psychiatric hospitalization. The level of social disadaptation of the EPIC clients is evidenced by the fact that only two were employed at the time of admission and 53% had no income whatsoever. The majority of the remainder received welfare, social security, or VA benefits.

Regardless of their previous levels of pathology or disadaptation, EPIC clients are viewed by the program as people with strengths and weaknesses, with innate worth, dignity, and rights. Starting with an assumption of competency, clients are encouraged to build on their strengths and to learn to solve their problems. The focus is on social rehabilitation including life management training, socialization-recreation programming, and individual, group and family counseling. . . .

The program offers considerable structure and support. Clients received an average of 25.2 planned counseling/therapy sessions per week (9.9 group; 15.3 individual). They also participated in an average of 6.3 social-recreation programs a week. Clients were seen by the . . . staff psychiatrist nearly once per week on the average. Medications are utilized as part of the therapeutic regime but at the lowest doses possible to bring about abatement of psychotic symptoms. A total of 67.4% of clients received medication during their entire EPIC residency, and 12.4% were not treated with psychoactive medication.

In examining the experience of the 89 EPIC clients discharged in the second fiscal year, it was found that 51% showed definite improvement, and 18% showed slight improvement in functioning as shown by improvement in global impairment scores and by discharges to settings in the community requiring higher levels of independent functioning. Of the EPIC clients who demonstrated no significant progress, a majority were relatively brief admissions where motivation for treatment and commitment to program participation were minimal. Difficulties common to this group included a lack of stabilization on medications prior to entry, an unwillingness to comply with medication as part of treatment, the presence of severe psychotic symptoms requiring rehospitalization, or a tendency toward street drug abuse. . . .

The experience of the EPIC program during its initial two years of operation indicates that short-term residential treatment in an open, structured program provides a cost-effective alternative to continued hospitalization.

While this organizational self-portrait no doubt puts on its best official face, it is useful to orient us to the organization's ideology, types and frequency of clinical practices, and some demographic and other social characteristics of its clients. The account also frankly acknowledges that most people have made most if not all of the stops in the psychiatric system before admission to EPIC. The report does not mention, however, that most EPIC residents continue to make these stops in their post-EPIC careers (which for over one-third of residents includes EPIC itself).

Organization Roles

The attempt to understand how psychiatric reality is built up must start with the formal organizational roles, "psychiatric staff" and "labeled psychotic." Constructionists see roles as analytic resumes of inventive interaction among people. Accordingly, roles may blur (or even disappear) at times. Nonetheless, each formal role carries with it explicit and implicit expectations based on official organizational status.

According to the *Annual Report*, the central role expectation for labeled psychotics at EPIC is "motivation for treatment," which is indicated mainly by cooperation with staff directives. Some key aspects of this role follow (cf. Parsons 1951, 1975; Friedson 1970; Fabrega 1972):

1. Admission that one is mentally ill (assuming the sick role).
2. Seeking help for this illness by attending group therapy and individual counseling sessions.
3. Taking drugs prescribed by the staff psychiatrist to abate symptoms.
4. Providing at least minimally for one's self-care, e.g., hygiene and grooming, as part of mental health.
5. Doing assigned household chores as part of healthy adaptation to everyday life.
6. Compliance with the program schedule, e.g., bedtimes and approved absences, as part of healthy adaptation.

The staff also have role expectations based upon formal organizational status. There are 12 regular staff positions at EPIC:

1. *Program supervisor:* S/he functions as overall administrator and clinical supervisor. The program supervisor works with the staff psychiatrist and underlying clinical staff to plan treatment, coordinate staff training, and act as liaison to the outside community.

2. *Staff psychiatrist:* The psychiatrist conducts diagnostic interviews, consults with staff on treatment issues, and prescribes and monitors the use of psychiatric drugs. S/he also oversees "psychological consults"—weekly staff meetings where the progress and prognosis of each client is discussed.

3. *Therapeutic team leader:* In essence a social worker, this person plans and implements therapy and counseling sessions, assesses clients' progress in treatment, and oversees "case management," i.e., placing clients in jobs (if possible) and shelter after discharge from EPIC. S/he also supervises underlying staff as de facto "clinical director."

4. *Residence manager:* This person oversees meals, transportation, and the general maintenance of the facility.

5. *Administrative assistant:* She is responsible for routine clerical tasks.

6. *Mental health workers:* These staff directly implement clinical activities and monitor all other aspects of clients' daily routine.

The Physical Setting

Outwardly EPIC does not look like a psychiatric facility. One walks up a concrete walkway to the entrance of an ordinary California ranch-style house in a typical middle-class suburban neighborhood. Only railroad tracks cut this suburban ambience, as trains streak past the left side of the house.

In front of the house near the entrance is an overgrown hedge. If one follows this hedge around the left side of the house, one finds that it encloses a half-acre yard that includes volleyball net, patio furniture, and lawn chairs. On nice days, staff and residents may be found playing volleyball or talking.

Upon entering the front door, one finds oneself in the "reception area"—a tiny office where the administrative assistant greets prospective residents and visitors. On the rear wall a large medicine cabinet juts from ill-fitting paneling. To the right a picture window scans the parking lot. To the left of the medicine cabinet a door opens into the larger office of the program supervisor where weekly psychological consults and staff meetings are held.

A large Dutch door opens from the reception area to the residents' recreation room. In fact, this door is the major physical border separating exclusively staff territory ("the office") from that shared by staff and residents. Most often the top half of the door is open and the bottom half closed. One often finds a resident leaning over it talking to a staff person in the office. During frequent staff retreats from residents, however, both halves are closed.

Passing through this door to the recreation room, one finds a pool table, two easy chairs, a couch, a small stereo, and a bookcase jammed with board games and reading material (mostly supermarket fare). Freewheeling discussions and horseplay often break out among residents here, and the stereo not infrequently blares through the closed Dutch door, demanding staff's attention.

A door opens from the recreation room into the Therapeutic team leader's office. This narrow, trailerlike room looks like it was forcibly wedged between the reception area and program supervisor's office. Two couches line the walls, and at the rear of the room is the team leader's desk, behind which a picture window looks out on the yard. Individual residents often enter this room to talk with the team leader about clinical and other matters.

The other end of the recreation room opens into the main living area. This large room no doubt was once the combined living and dining rooms for a typical suburban family, and it still functions similarly.

Three large couches, a few occasional chairs and tables, and a TV fill this area. Two picture windows face the walkway and parking lot at the front of the house. Numerous posters and pictures dot the walls. They include inspirational wall hangings—"This is the first day of the rest of your life," "If life gives you lemons make lemonade"—and the eclectic productions of residents in "art therapy"groups. Most clinical and leisure activities occur here, including "group therapy," TV-watching, meals, just "hanging out," talking—or even napping on a couch.

The dining area has two large wooden dining tables placed end to end and circled by an eclectic group of straight-backed chairs. A large lunch counter divides this area from the kitchen, where each meal is prepared by two residents supervised by a staff person. This suburban kitchen has the usual major appliances and culinary devices.

A door from the living area opens into the back of the house, where four bedrooms accommodate two residents each (when the house if full). Two bathrooms and a pay telephone are also in this "backstage" area. Tucked away near one of the bedrooms is a small room containing just a desk and love seat. The staff psychiatrist conducts diagnostic interviews here.

Concluding this brief tour, one exits at the rear of the house onto a winding path leading to a smaller building. Dubbed the "bunkhouse" by natives, this structure houses three bedrooms and a bathroom, and as a relatively isolated spot is seen by residents as the most desirable room assignment. Staff agree, and reserve these rooms for residents whom they see as "least sick" and therefore best able to handle greater independence from supervision.

Field Methods

The research at EPIC took place over one and one-half years (January 1983 to August 1984), during which I was a participant observer in all aspects of the setting for a few days a week, and for the first six months of the study also worked part-time on the night shift. (Prior to becoming a sociologist,

I had worked for over eight years in paraprofessional capacities in a wide variety of psychiatric settings.) At first, "natives" (i.e., staff and residents) who did not know me were suspicious of my presence. Labeled psychotics often viewed me as a psychiatrist. Throughout the study I worked to disabuse them of this notion (with mixed results). Both groups at first feared that as an "expert" I would make them cogs in some conceptual system—whether psychiatric or sociological. As Greg, a staff person, succinctly put it after our interview:

> I enjoyed our talk. I thought it would be more about the mental health system and general sociological patterns than personal stuff. I was pleasantly surprised.

Maintaining access to a setting is an ongoing process of eliciting natives' trust and cooperation. To do so is necessary because the participants have the power to shut the study down. All field researchers face, implicitly or explicitly, the inevitable "What's in it for me?" question of denizens.

Beside proving trustworthy by keeping confidences and protecting participants' anonymity, I offered "amenities" in return for cooperation. I always lent a sympathetic ear to staff's complaints about the job—an important source of data. I also offered to write recommendations for jobs or school that named them as "research assistants" (which, indeed, they were). At times I showed staff anonymous fragments from interview transcripts and invited commentary. Although they rarely took me up on these offers, staff reciprocated my overtures by informing me of activities about which I otherwise would have remained ignorant, e.g., impromptu meetings and household "crises."

As for residents, for the most part just my listening without judgment to their personal stories seemed enough for them. I also offered them recommendations, and unlike staff they took me up on this offer. On occasion I ran errands for residents or bought them sundry items like candy or cigarettes (which no doubt reinforced their typically awful nutritional habits).

My basic approach in the field was to sit around EPIC and casually talk with natives as they went about their activities. These talks ranged from passing comments to bull sessions lasting over an hour, and often involved two or more people. Out of these talks I arranged private and confidential individual interviews. The typical length of these interviews was about two hours. In all situations I carried a tape recorder and a stenographer's notebook, and used them roughly equally to record events (see "Observer Effects" below).

My choices of interviewees are not based on formal sampling criteria. Of the 120 diagnosed psychotics who passed through EPIC during this period, 41 were interviewed. The labeled psychotics include 24 men and 17 women (about 60 percent of admissions were men), and their mean age is 29. Fourteen were diagnosed as schizophrenic, 16 as manic depressives, and 11 as having schizoaffective disorders.[8] All regular and most part-time staff employed during the period of the research (inclucing 2 psychiatrists), plus 1 student volunteer, were interviewed—28 in all. The staff include 13 men and 15 women (EPIC hiring policies emphasize gender balance), and their mean age is 31.

Fictitious names are used to protect participants' anonymity and confidentiality. References to persons by name are preceded by the codes "(S)" for "staff" and "(R)" for "labeled psychotic," unless the person's organizational role is clear in context. Exceptions to this procedure are Drs. Williams (or "Dr. W") and Ogden (or "Dr. O"), who are always referred to as such (or as "DR"), and myself (referred to as "BL").

Formal interviews at first retained the completely open-ended format of the informal talks, but over time I began to notice that staff and residents alike often brought up unsolicited personal problems or strange experiences. I noticed too that both groups frequently used psychiatric diagnostic language in relation to these experiences. I became particularly interested in what appeared to be the staff's seemingly equal use of these terms in light of their obligation to be "healthy" role models in the interest of rehabilitation. In fact, this latter development would become the basis of the study.

This study began with my general interest in the effects of the psychiatric ideology of psychosis on residents in a psychiatric setting, but after much thought about staff's use of psychiatric terms, the central issue shifted to the extent to which this ideology constructed the staff's social world. The key goals became to document the impact of this ideology on staff and the interpersonal strategies they develop in relation to this impact. Accordingly, four interwoven empirical questions upon which this study now hinges took shape:

1. Does the staff's job to detect symptoms of psychosis in their patients lead staff to apply these criteria to their own behavior (i.e., to self-label)?
2. If the staff apply the psychiatric ideology of psychosis to their own behavior, does this activity threaten their work roles?
3. Do the staff's constructions of their patient's behavior as symptoms of psychosis rebound to threaten their *own* self-definitions as competent people?
4. If the staff consistently self-label and are so threatened in the ways indicated, what interpersonal strategies do they use to resist the threat?

Thus this study addresses how staff ironically orient to labeled psychotics as role models, or "reverse role models." It mainly entails how staff attempt to keep personal problems arising in the context of their work with labeled psychotics from becoming a *social* problem as evidence of "mental illness."

When I first noticed the pattern of staff's use of psychiatric terms for their own experiences, the theme of reverse role modeling had not yet emerged. Staff's use of these terms, however, decisively influenced my developing the following interview question from which this theme was largely to develop: "Have you ever had experiences (feelings, thoughts, behavior) that you would call unusual compared to how you usually experience your life?" I then asked each person to describe these self-defined unusual experiences as specifically and fully as possible.

My use of "unusual experiences" in this question was intended as a personally and socially relative, entirely context-dependent construction. Accordingly, I was careful to explain to each interviewee that s/he ought to use his or her own life as the yardstick for answering it. For example, Jane may perceive her behavior in some setting as being unusual compared to her usual behavior in that same setting. Or Jane may see her behavior in a setting as usual for her, and only unusual in comparison with her view of Cleo's behavior in the same setting.

However, it must be stressed that, while this question became an important benchmark in the study, the interviews remained mostly freewheeling, even rambling affairs. Interviewees were encouraged to coauthor our talk with concerns they brought to it. Interviews were living events, never constrained to travel only on the rails of my agenda. Here is an example from my interview with (S) Melissa:

We enter Dr. Williams' office together. Melissa sits down across the office from me. She remains silent for quite some time, her eyes averted.

Melissa: I don't know if I can concentrate on any questions [She is eight months pregnant and the weather is very hot.] I feel "spacy."

Bruce: That's OK. Let's just sit here. I don't want to impose anything on you.

Melissa: If you're sure that's what you want.

Bruce: Well, it's the more real part of how I see this work—meeting you where you're coming from.

Melissa: Because I think I can answer whatever questions you want me to if I really want to, if I won't be so lazy, a little bit more self-disciplined—which is maybe what I expect from a lot of clients too—to pull themselves back from 'spaciness.' When it gets in the way of managing their lives, I think they need to be brought back. [Long pause.] But this is incredible, what's happening. [Pause.] I thought *you* would be getting stuff from this interview, but I'm getting more.

Bruce: What do you mean?

Melissa: I mean I haven't really thought of it being like this before, but it's true. We're doing this together. [Pause.] Maybe I shouldn't pull clients back from their experiences so fast.

Melissa makes demands on herself that she be more "self-disciplined" in answering what she imagines are my preconceived questions. But when I do not reinforce her demand that she be an object of my questions, and instead encourage her to be herself in what she calls her "spacy" condition, the border between interviewer and interviewee starts to dissolve. She sees not only that we are mutually constructing the interview, but also that she and her patients similarly coauthor psychiatric reality. And by empathetically taking the role of the residents—her own pregnant, "spacy" condition likened to their "spaciness"—she begins to dissolve the border between psychiatric staff as subject and labeled psychotic as work object. In her words, "We're doing this [interview/psychiatric reality/life] together."

Thus I am aware that this study was jointly produced by the natives of this setting and myself. This standpoint enabled me to succeed, for the most part, in providing ample room for the subjective agenda of each interviewee. Nonetheless, the reader will discover that I am mostly absent from the text of this study—save as its authorial voice. And though I let many native voices speak, I also know that this centralization of narrative authority does not fully avoid imposing my interpretive standpoint on their descriptions. My subsequent ethnographic work will attempt to embody a more radical decentralization of authorship. (See "Endnote on Critical Ethnography" in Chapter 6 for further discussion of this issue.)

Besides the informal talks and formal interviews, my materials derive also from participant observation in three major organizational contexts: psychological consults, group therapies, and diagnostic interviews. I attended 16 psychological consults. These sessions are weekly staff conferences (out of earshot of patients) in which each patient's clinical progress and prognosis is discussed. I also attended 18 group therapy sessions, in which staff and patients explore patients' problems in living. Finally, I observed 14 diagnostic interviews in which, as the name indicates, the staff psychiatrist clinically evaluates newly admitted patients.

Observer Effects

During the study I was careful to notice any signs of participants' discomfort with my procedures of notetaking and tape recording. Objections were rare. The vast majority of natives appeared to accustom themselves very quickly to these devices. Like furniture, they were virtually ignored. I met the occasional complaint by stopping the procedure, and only later sneaking off to a private spot to jot a note or two.

This issue of the effects of the researcher and his tools on social phenomena involves the important and controversial sociological issue of observer effects, or what is also called "reactivity" (Rosenthal 1966; Rosenthal and Jacobson 1968). The goal of removing or reducing subjective influence on social research as "bias"—like so much static interfering with an otherwise clear signal—is in my judgment not only misguided but impossible. This pillar of positivistic method—sociologist as detached observer—needs to crumble along with the rest of its nineteenth-century architecture.

Sociologist cannot remove subjective influence by fiat. Instead, we ought to admit that our subjective vantage points (including faith in objective reality) create the substance of our studies, and take care to meet our obligation to reveal our moral and political commitments—to declare "whose side we are on" (Becker 1967). As researchers, our individual realities dance with the social worlds of natives as part of the gorgeous surfeit of subjectivity to be celebrated, not banished. From these steps comes social reality.

I have tried to create a rigorously grounded study (Glaser and Strauss 1967), but never an objective one. And if what I see from my vantage point is not what you see in your light, I am sorry. But I neither despair of nor begrudge you your view of matters, for no doubt each of us from our different perches can take flight.

Notes

1. Weber defines power as "the probabililty that one actor within a social relationship will be in a position to carry out his own will despite resistance" (Weber 1958:183). He also defines authority (or domination—the German *Herrschaft* may be translated either way) as "the probability that a command with a given specific content will be obeyed by a given group of persons." And Weber defines agreement with one's subordination, i.e., legitimation, and crucial to any sociology of deviance, as part of ongoing social convention: "A system of order will be called convention so far as its validity is externally guaranteed by the probability that deviation from it within a given social group will result in a relatively general and practically significant reaction of disapproval" (Weber 1966:127).

2. I must emphasize, however, that this framework is *not* intended as an all-inclusive schema through which all social problems must "evolve," but rather illustrates the typical empirical logic of many social problems. Also, certainly groups can and do enter into claims-making activity at any point in the process—

sometimes not getting beyond stage 1 before such activity aborts. At the other end, some groups from the outset reject the ability or willingness of current agencies and institutions to address their concerns, and thus launch their contention as attempts to form "counterinstitutions." In fact, the latter emphasis is at the center of my critical approach.

3.   Watson here cites Israel (1971:346), who in turn was citing G. Radnitsky's (1970) *Contemporary Schools of Metascience.*

4.   I use this term, first coined by Thomas Szasz (1961), as a descriptive ordinary expression that neither degrades the people so troubled nor is loaded with psychiatric ideological baggage.

5.   My brief overview of the politics of community psychiatry is indebted to Henry W. Vandenburgh's (1979) interesting and well-researched unpublished paper, "Critical Theory and Mental Health and Illness."

6.   In some California counties of seventh stop, a "crisis facility," also constitutes part of the system. However, many such crisis facilities were closed during the 1980s for lack of funding—largely because they have no potential for profit, as do admissions to proprietary hospitals. East Lake County's crisis facility closed in 1980.

7.   Excerpted from *Annual Report 1981, 82,* Psychiatric Intervention Community Services, East Lake County, California. pp. 7–9.

8.   I shall not outline here the psychiatric model of the other major psychosis, "manic depression" (or more technically, "bipolar disorder"). A very colorful and descriptively accurate portrait of its alleged behavioral features is presented in Erving Goffman's *Insanity of Place* (1971).

Chapter 2

BORDER CROSSING

Crossing the Border

This study begins with the point of departure for the labeled-psychotic career at EPIC, that is, the diagnostic interview. Excerpts from three interviews represent processes typical of all fourteen observed.

The first interview begins with staff psychiatrist Dr. Ogden asking Terry to "tell me something about yourself." Terry answers as follows:

> [Terry's voice is brightly high-pitched, though she speaks slowly and with a wary hesitancy. Her eyes dart to and fro between Dr. O, myself, and the floor.] I had lots of temporary jobs with Manpower last year, and I was a flight attendant for six and a half years before that.

Terry presents herself as a conscientious worker. Dr. O continues:

> [His voice is soft, gentle, and sweet—but with a singsong inflection like that often heard when adults address children or the elderly.] You're not saying much about your personal life. This is all your work life. Did you have a personal life—or do you just shut that out?

Dr. O admonishes Terry for not mentioning a personal life. He perhaps also implies that she talks about her work history in order to avoid poor or nonexistent personal relations. In any case, Terry replies:

> In Torrance I had lots of friends. I had friends coming out of my ears. My best friend . . . was the homecoming queen. But I had maybe five friends where I was raised. They knew me all my life.

Terry's claim to have had many friends no doubt addresses Dr. O's implicit view that a normal life includes friends and, conversely, that the absence of friends may be symptomatic of mental illness. He replies as follows:

[He has been turning pages of Terry's file distractedly as she speaks. He stops here and there to study a page, and occasionally looks up at her.] But that was in high school in Torrance. What about here in Lakeside?

While not contesting the early friendships, Dr. O seems to suggest a decline since Terry's youth, the context of her claim. Terry responds accordingly:

But in the airlines and college I still had friends. I worked for the airlines six and a half years. So you've been asking for my life's story, and I was giving you a general outline. If I could spend a day I could give you every nook and cranny.

Terry protests the implicit challenge to her social competence in Dr. O's remarks on her personal life. By claiming to have had friends at work and college (the educational reference being added evidence of competence), Terry serves notice to the doctor that she views herself as a competent adult. She thereby resists what she sees as Dr. O's invasion of her life ("every nook and cranny") to prove otherwise.

Dr. O: Looking at your chart I hear about a different person than I see here
          today.
Terry: Yeah, I am.

While apparently conceding that Terry is presenting herself competently now, Dr. O refers to her file, which, he says, tells a "different" story:

Dr. O: Apparently you were quite out of it when you got to the hospital.
Terry: This last time. [Her voice lowers and trails off as she looks at the floor.]

Dr. O openly refers to Terry as having been "out of it," that is, mentally ill. Her past competence so discredited, Terry drops her eyes to the floor and her voice to a whisper (gestures themselves sometimes called symptoms). And by conceding "this last time" to Dr. O's characterization, Terry implicitly hopes to save any other times from being so constructed. He continues:

Dr. O: The previous time too. How much of a memory can you allow yourself
          of those times?
Terry: I don't remember any of those times [inaudible] last time.
Dr. O: Would you talk about this time?
Terry: I don't care to.
Dr. O: Did you have bad feelings during this time?

Terry: [Haltingly. Well [her voice grows suddenly loud and angry] I don't remember really enough to tell you. [As she makes fleeting eye contact with Dr. O, her voice trails off to a whisper, and her gaze again fixes on the floor.] I, [she stammers] I couldn't go into detail if I tried. There was so much happening in a short period of time. It happened so fast. It's hard to sit down and say this. I, [she stammers] I couldn't. [Her voice breaks off in silence.]

As Dr. O digs into her past over her objections, Terry starts to protest, but then becomes silent and outwardly unresponsive. Dr. O then goes on to probe her alleged history of drinking. Suddenly she blurts that she used to drink "like everybody else," but no longer does so due to her religious beliefs. With that, Dr. O leans forward, staring intently at Terry, and asks:

Dr. O: Have you taken your religion seriously?
Terry: Uhh, [she stammers] I think I've always been religious. I think now more than ever.

Dr. O does not probe Terry's reply, but tells me after the interview that Terry has been hospitalized for "religious delusions." He then brings up Terry's relationship with her parents:

Dr. O: Have your parents at times yelled and screamed at you?
Terry: Yes.
Dr. O: Over what sorts of issues?
Terry: [She laughs for the first and only time, then blurts loudly and sharply] Where I've been wrong and they've been right! Tell me what's right!
Dr. O: It's pretty, [pauses] I, [stammers] I . . .
Terry: [She cuts him off sharply.] Like staying on my medication! [Her voice quiets again.] Well, it's never been anything major. There were times they yelled at me—were trying to help me.

Here Terry confronts both parental and medical attempts to "help" her by enforcing the "right" course of conduct or treatment. "They" (whether parents or doctor) are implicitly always "right," she asserts sarcastically, whereas she (as child and patient) is always "wrong."

Terry's forceful challenge to Dr. O momentarily stops him in his tracks, reducing his smug delivery to a stammer. Dr. O seems threatened by this sudden, albeit brief turning of the tables in the doctor/patient transaction, whereby Terry assumes the dominant role. In any case, Terry implicitly sees Dr. O's role as the twin of parental authority—family treatment coming full circle in clinical treatment. At this point Dr. O ends the interview. After Terry leaves, Dr. O tells me that she suffers from a schizoaffective disorder.

Staff psychiatrist Dr. Williams begins the next interview by asking Janice why her "stresses" build up to the point of hospitalization. She answers as follows:

> I was the landlady of the house. I took no drugs and took care of my baby for three years. But people [living in the house] didn't pay rent and they stole my welfare checks. I want a cleaner and better house for my baby without roaches.

Janice presents herself as a responsible landlady and parent who was victimized by dishonest and irresponsible tenants. And she projects a future goal of a better house and associates.

> *Dr. W:* Are there any other emotional illnesses in the family?
> *Janice:* My mom died of cancer when I was ten. It took five years. I knew since seven I had to take care of my dad, brother—the whole house. My dad remarried when I was seventeen, but my stepmom didn't like me and kicked me out of the house.

Janice ignores Dr. W's question, which assumes that she has an emotional illness (perhaps among "others" in the family). Instead, she talks of tragically losing her mother, and implies that as a child she nonetheless competently handled the adult burden of caring for her family until the conflict with her stepmother (over control of the household?). Dr. W then asks:

> Do you have any other emotional problems?

He constructs Janice's social account of her troubles as evidence of an "emotional problem." Janice replies as follows:

> Once I overdosed at 14. I drank a lot of beer and someone put something in it, trying to kill me. But I don't do drugs anymore. I wanted to have a healthy baby. Lots of young people experiment. I went to the hospital for two months.

Janice again claims that her hospitalization was the result of victimization—this time being drugged against her will. She also contends that after a period of (implicitly normal) experimentation with drugs she became a drug-free and responsible parent.

But by answering Dr. W's question about her "emotional problems" with this story of drug overdose (voluntary or not) leading to hospitalization for two months, Janice acknowledges his psychiatric definition of her situation. Dr. W responds as follows:

Dr. W: Why so long?
Janice: To get me back together again.

Dr. W's reaction to the length of her stay, given that the mean psychiatric hospitalization is less than two weeks, suggests his belief that Janice is quite mentally ill. And Janice's claim that she needed this long a stay to "get me back together again" logically concedes a prior "untogetherness" (illness) from which to recover. Dr. W probes accordingly:

Dr. W: What do you mean back together again?
Janice: My brainwaves were like this. [Janice throws her elbows out, points her index fingers together, and moves her hands up and down methodically and rigidly.]

Janice's gesture implicitly applies the psychiatric disease model of a biologically dysfunctional mind to her behavior. It bespeaks her acceptance that she is mentally ill. Just then Dr. W ends the interview. But while leaving the room, Janice offers the following:

I was seven, and my mom was sick and in pain for back cancer. The doctors just kept giving her codeine while her cancer spread to her brain. My dad then bought me a horse after she died, and someone poisoned it. This was too much for a little girl to handle.

Throughout the interview Dr. W disregards Janice's attempts to provide social explanations for her personal problems. And though she acquiesces to his psychiatric model, in the end she again depicts her private difficulties as socially intelligible. Alongside apparent criticism of the medical treatment given to her mother (and implicitly herself), she suggests that social misfortune underlies her personal troubles and, indeed, would be "too much for [any] little girl to handle." Dr. W concludes that Janice is suffering from schizophrenia.

The last interview concerns Efrem, whose file shows no stays in psychiatric settings until shortly before this interview. Dr. W begins by asking Efrem if he was hospitalized before.

Efrem: Yes, I was in Napa [state hospital] four months ago, but I don't want to talk about it now.
Dr. W: How were you feeling then?
Efrem: [His voice and bearing, at first quiet, languid, detached, and distracted—if marked by a flicker of surliness—grows louder now, smoldering with barely contained anger.] I executed people in 1968 in [Viet] Nam who were badly broken up. My wife and three kids died in an auto crash while I was there. Who wouldn't snap?

Probed over his objection, Efrem moves quickly to provide Dr. W with a social explanation of his troubles. He suggests that given the same circumstances, anybody would have responded as he did ("who wouldn't snap?")

Dr. W: Did you ever try to hurt yourself?
Efrem: No, I just flipped a car once—but that was an accident.
Dr. W: You seem nervous. How can we help you relax?
Efrem: I need to be less uptight, but I don't get uptight in a violent way. I can't put it into words.

Efrem rejects Dr. W's probe for suicidal acts (symptoms) by claiming that he accidentally overturned a car once. By so doing he again meets Dr. W's search for evidence of irrationality with a rational account of his behavior—accidents happen to everybody. Dr. W then seems to imply that Efrem's "nervousness" is a personality trait having little to do with the present situation (for one thing, being questioned over his objections). Nonetheless, Efrem frankly acknowledges emotional turmoil and his need to be "less uptight," but quickly denies any propensity for violence. This unsolicited remark perhaps suggests guilt over wartime activities ("execut[ing] people" leading to a pathos beyond words)—or maybe just veiled sarcasm at his felt violation at being probed despite his objections.

Dr. W: [He leafs through his file on Efrem.] It says here you were living in the woods before coming to EPIC. Isn't living in the woods kind of aimless?
Efrem: [He pauses, staring dreamily or vacantly out the window.] Yeah, but I got a lot of reading done.
Dr. W: You need help to get back into life—get a job?
Efrem: I don't like idleness, but I don't like jobs, either.
Dr. W: Do you want to try to get direction in your life?
Efrem: I want to learn to be independent. It makes me nervous to be dependent. Outsiders have more control.

Dr. W calls Efrem's living in the woods "aimless" (His "aimful" career as soldier goes unquestioned.) Efrem's distracted staring out the window and sarcastic comments on reading and jobs suggest resistance to this implicit judgment that his life is disordered (and, therefore, that he is disordered). Further, his desire to be independent and his being "nervous" about dependence suggest the fear of loss of control of his life to "outsiders" as the source of his troubles. After all, his soldier role abroad and tragedy at home mean nothing if not loss of control over his social circumstances—a loss ironically again in the making here as the source of his resistance.

Efrem's hard experience has led him to confront Dr. W's implicit model of a normal life: In this model, job (even if killing as soldier) = direction = social legitimacy = normal life. Conversely, no job (even if peaceful and active as reader) = aimlessness = social illegitimacy = abnormal life. For Efrem this equation has never added up.

Dr. W: Do you sometimes feel outsiders have more control?
Efrem: [In a surly tone of voice,] No, I have no paranoid fantasies about secret police—nobody is out to get me.

Efrem tells me elsewhere that a doctor in the state hospital told him that he had a "paranoid-schizophrenic" disorder. That perhaps explains his use of the term "paranoid" here as an attempt to head off its being applied again. But Efrem's prior remark that dependence made him nervous because "outsiders have more control" is a key diagnostic indicator of the paranoid part of the alleged disorder. It probably leads Dr. W to repeat Efrem's comment about control as a probe for verification. In any case, making this claim to a psychiatric authority ironically calls forth the application of the term. And Efrem's explicit use of the term "paranoid" to deny anybody is "out to get" him unwittingly jumps directly into its line of fire. He is thereby "gotten." There is no need for "secret police."

Dr. W: Do you lose touch with reality?
Efrem: No, but in my head I need more space.

Dr. W, with Efrem's file in hand, probably is checking out the "schizophrenic" half of Efrem's diagnosis in the state hospital. In any case, the question indicates a probe for Efrem's orientation to reality—whether he is deluded or hallucinates, key diagnostic indicators of schizophrenia. Denying he loses touch with reality, Efrem's comment about needing "more space" again resists the ongoing search here for evidence of his social and psychological incompetence. Efrem is anything but guarded and suspicious (other key diagnostic indicators of paranoia) in the interview. Raw and open with his feelings and candid—if confrontational—in his views, he is ironically not self-protective enough.

Dr. W ends the interview and Efrem leaves the office. Dr. W then turns to me and asks:

Dr. W: Do you think he's psychotic?
BL: I'd rather not offer an opinion. As a researcher, I want to stay out of the picture as far as possible in your interviews.
Dr. W: [Somewhat sharply,] But you've worked in the field and have some clinical picture.

BL: That [Efrem's account of his war experiences and family tragedy] seems like it might be enough to cause what he's going through, without going back into his family history, which he was sketchy about.

Dr. W: Well, he's an interesting guy. [Long pause.] But a healthy person would after a period of grief integrate that stuff after awhile—and he wouldn't need two more hospitalizations.

BL: [I nod ever so slightly.]

This is the only time during 14 interviews that Dr. W asks for my opinion before rendering his diagnostic verdict. I have no doubt that the poignancy of Efrem's social circumstances leads Dr. W to hesitate before making his decision (though such hesitancy was curiously lacking in the interviews of women like Janice and Maude, whose circumstances strike me as similarly poignant). I answer honestly about not wanting to influence unduly what would have happened had I not been there.

However, Dr. W shows some annoyance at my reluctance to offer my "clinical picture," which in any case cannot be rendered so neatly in the mutually exclusive categories, psychotic/nonpsychotic. When pressed by the doctor, I offer a more social explanation, which backs Efrem's claim to competence and thus "depsychoticizes" his situation. Dr. W seems to give my position some thought, but then opts for his psychiatric definition of Efrem's situation. In order to maintain my access to these interviews, I nod assent. Efrem is diagnosed "paranoid schizophrenic." We have just crossed the border.

Caught in the Net

No strangers to diagnostic interviews, the vast majority of EPIC residents have been hospitalized, most more than once, as part of the circuitous psychiatric system sketched in Chapter 1: from home, to hospital, to "community" (i.e., halfway house, cheap hotel, or the streets), back to the hospital, and so on. (R) Shran characterizes this situation as follows:

It's like the 'patienthood/staffhood syndrome.' It's an interesting theory: Patients and staff perpetuate each other. The doctor says, 'you've got problems, we'll help you with them.' The patient provides a place for the staff when they keep coming back. It just keeps going around in circles. . . . When I first found out about this stuff, I wanted to scream.

Shran tersely summarizes the essential pattern of the psychiatric system and, finding no exit, he "wanted to scream." In this system the mental hospital, the setting from which most EPIC residents are directly recruited, is the point of origin of the labeled psychotic career. The character of the mental hospital requires elaboration.

For all its often unpleasant and sometimes painful features of social control (see below), the hospital is at least physically safe, warm, and dry, provides three meals daily (albeit with drug "condiments"), has linen service, hot and cold running water, and a housekeeping staff to clean up after one. As (S) Kris puts it:

> It's [the hospital] like home. When things get heavy, some of us [staff] go to wives or family, get drunk, or stay alone. Some [labeled psychotics] go to the hospital—because that's where the juice is for them. Society is not creating a niche for them. The niche these people have is the mental health system, as weird as it may be and as much as they may hate it. In some ways it's like a church. It's a very accepting niche where you don't have to do much, a kind of catchall—also a garbage can. I think a lot of people are blown out.

An institutional mother of sorts, the hospital is a reliable and secure home base where "blown-out" people at least always find paid caretakers and known friends and associates in the same "garbage can" or "church"—depending on your vantage point. The alternative—living in the "community"—often means enduring a run-down hotel with urine-stained, odorous hallways, cockroaches and other vermin, unreliable or even dangerous associates, and irregular meals of poor nutritional value (when available, given no or low incomes and rooms without kitchens). And this is to be preferred over the unforgiving streets.

But what about the original families? EPIC residents comment:

Samuel: I'm emotional, hurting, frustrated, confused, and lonely. I got a raw deal in life. I'm the only unsuccessful one in my family. My sisters finished college at 16, I quit in ninth grade—I've been on my own for a long time with no support.

Maude: Both parents were alcoholics and finally died . . . when I was about 12. I was in 4 or 5 foster homes as a teenager, and was molested twice by my foster fathers.

Kate: I was the middle child. And I look back now and realize I was a battered child. My father made welts on my legs because I wouldn't talk. I've been spit on by my father, and my mother mistreated me badly.

Maureen: My mom was negative about giving money, was pejorative, mostly insane—a nasty son of a bitch to talk to. I got tons of criticism, a big influence on my life. My family turns away from my problems, no support. My family brought me to my knees.

Simone: I was taking [drugs] . . . valium, speed, and was drinking. I was
            leaving my son with my parents since . . . I got my divorce . . . I
            mess up. I was always fighting with my dad. He was always telling
            me what, how, why, and where, because I had no other place to go.
Eddie: I had a strict family, a fearful childhood. I know the 'whys'—a lack of
            love and affection from my parents and strict punishment. Sex was
            a dirty word. To express my feelings, I set the house on fire to burn
            away the unloved atmosphere. I was 6. "Southern hospitality" and
            southern punishment.

This collective portrait shows the families of EPIC residents to be
fraught with conflict, abuse, instability, and drug and alcohol problems.
Caught between the devil of original families, cheap hotels, board and
care homes, and the deep blue sea of the streets, it is little wonder that
most labeled psychotics, after initial (often forced) hospitalizations, come
to choose the hospital or EPIC as "home." We turn now to look more
closely at the social worlds of the psychiatric hospital and EPIC.

Nowhere to Hide

Admitting to considerable emotional turmoil in their everyday lives,
residents speak of coming to EPIC searching for support. (R) Earl talks
about his experience:

> Staff go out of their way to let me know about things I do that work against
> me. For instance, I used to bust into conversations and cut everyone off, and
> stand real close. It made everybody uptight about me. Staff helped me see
> that I did this because I felt no good and that no one would listen to me if I
> didn't force them to. . . . I do better here than at a party, not because of the
> structure, but because staff start closing in and zeroing in on something and
> tell me what to do. [He pauses.] The staff try to help me too much—
> sometimes the system tries to help too much.

Earl is typical of residents in depicting much altruism among staff—
their genuine desire to be helpful. While fully acknowledging staff's
concern for his welfare, and that this interest is helpful in some important
respects, Earl also shows the typical ambiguity among residents regarding the nature of staff's involvement. His words suggest some discomfort
with the scrutiny of his actions by the staff. In fact, his phrases "closing
in" and "zeroing in" have an almost military cast to them. And his final
complaint about staff's overhelpfulness abstracted as "the system" suggests that he feels boxed in by psychiatry as a bureaucratic mechanism.
(R) Kate comments:

Staff told me I was too sexual with the guys, but I wasn't—I mean I never did anything 'wrong' but be friendly and maybe flirt a little. Now I'm confused—I don't know how to channel it (my sexuality). Laying in bed in my room, I even got afraid to masturbate, and I did it before kindergarten.

Kate adds that she is always afraid that staff will find something she is doing "inappropriate" (the word most often used by staff to censure residents' behavior). Virtually all residents complain that staff monitor their behavior too closely. For example, most residents note that staff often will enter their rooms without knocking or awaiting a reply. Having their behavior probed without warning also disturbs many residents, who resent constant pressure to be "on" emotionally—ready to field staff questions aimed at correcting their lives. While most residents agree that EPIC is less severe than the hospital in this regard, they nonetheless point out that an intrusive surveillance constructs daily life in all the psychiatric settings they have experienced.

We turn now to the related issue of psychiatric drugs. (R) Teresa comments:

Mellaril [a phenothiazine drug] and lithium aren't that bad physically, and Mellaril relaxes me. I'm not 'zombied out' like with Thorazine [also a phenothiazine], and my jaw doesn't lock and I don't feel like I can't get comfortable, needing to pace all the time. But Mellaril breaks down my defenses. I wouldn't want to be on it if negotiating with the chancellor [college president]. If my defenses are broken down, I can be convinced to accept anything.

Teresa is positive about some of the drugs' calming effects. In fact most residents (73 percent, or 30 out of 41 in my interviews) say these drugs provide some relief from the painful anxiety and/or hellish imagery that they admit often overwhelm and terrorize them. But under their influence Teresa also feels vulnerable to control by anyone in authority, or—in a word—powerless. Having been a student political activist at the university, she is particularly wary of the drugs' potential as tools of social control and manipulation as part and parcel of the issue of invasive surveillance. (R) Nanette comments:

They [drugs] slow down and depress my moods immensely. When I don't take them, I'm aware, fast, speedy [she snaps her fingers], quick and bright. When I take them, I sleep, am drowsy, dizzy—more depressed—sleepy and dopey all the time. It's a doped up, unaware state of mind. It was very impure—I felt persecuted by drugs.

Unlike Teresa, Nanette has nothing positive to say about psychiatric drugs. While stopping short of feeling "persecuted," the vast majority of residents concur with her basic point about the drugs creating a "dopey," "sleepy," "unaware state of mind" (what Teresa and many others refer to as a zombielike state). Residents also consistently complain of weight gain (especially with lithium) and nausea in relation to the drugs. Further, virtually all residents on the drugs report having had, at some time, one or more of the following reactions: involuntary licking of lips, protruding tongue, eyes rolling back in the head, bouncing on balls of the feet, stiffness and tremors of torso and limbs, and other assorted muscular twitches and ticks.

With increased dosage and time on these drugs, these physiological symptoms multiply and intensify as expressive of *irreversible* damage to the central nervous system.[1] Worse, this condition, tardive dyskinesia, often does not show up until the drugs are stopped—ironically requiring more of the same drugs to remask the problem, thereby deepening it, and so on.

Finally, residents complain of negative social reactions to these drug-induced behaviors, which compound their problems as people labeled ill in the first place for behavior thought odd. In sum, "Club Med(ication)" is a trip few residents want to take. Dr. Williams speaks to this issue, using (R) Vern as an example:

> Vern [a young resident vehemently opposed to these drugs] is right to an extent. He feels the effects of medicine as somewhat negative. Most people do. It slows them down, slows their thinking down, makes their body feel different—heaviness and slowness—even if it benefits thinking. There are real problems with it for most people. That's one reason, other than in principle, people don't like to take it.

Dr. Williams joins residents in pointing to major problems with the drugs (though he does not mention tardive dyskinesia, and residents, while claiming some emotional benefits, rarely say that any of these drugs "benefits thinking"). But there is another issue bound up with the invasive character of these drugs, which for some residents has priority over the emotive and bodily aspects emphasized so far. Maureen comments:

> I went through this thing about God and people in heaven talking to me, which involved partly how we make our own hell, and that there is no hell. I'm still flipped about it. Then I was put on lithium and Stelazine [a phenothiazine] and it all faded. My mind got so fuzzy I couldn't stay in contact with people here or in heaven.

Some residents express misgivings or hostility toward what they see as chemical obstacles to their spiritual progress. They believe that their "unusual experiences," even while accompanied by emotional turmoil, bring positive or even reconstitutive lessons to their lives. (R) Vern, to whom Dr. Williams alluded to above, comments:

> I think it's an enslavement . . . to have to take medication [drugs]. I would like to be here at EPIC without medication, and one of the rules is that you can't be at EPIC without medication. I think medication is a drug like any other drug—it puts you in an altered state of consciousness you shouldn't necessarily be in. It's like hell—I feel like I hear lots of things and conversations on different levels of reality at once without drugs. I'm striving for spirituality, and EPIC isn't conducive to that.

And what of Vern's claims? As architects of social life, do we not create incredibly complex inner (psychological) and outer social worlds? Consulting my own life, I experience a kaleidoscopic, often cacophonous array of thoughts, feelings, sights, and sounds—"lots of things and conversations on different levels of reality at once" (analogous in cybernetics to an endless feedback loop). What if this plenitude were suddenly to contract to only a narrow and rigid band of experience? The personal threat I feel in contemplating such a condition greatly heightens my empathy with Vern.

For some residents this closure may bring blessed relief. But for others, who may have unhinged the door to the centerless dance of phenomena (perhaps to wondrous worlds beyond our reach), this change may indeed be "like hell"—a very grave loss. Psychiatric drugs may so constrict the range of experience that people like Vern feel "enslaved" by them. In any case, Maureen and Vern believe they have "broken through," or will break through, to more profound realities and self-understandings if drug free.

Thus residents indicate that psychiatric drugs are an integral part of what most suggest is an invasive scrutiny by staff in psychiatric settings. However, drugs as a major tool of the psychiatric enterprise make up but one component of the concepts and practices that attempt to reshape residents' social realities. (R) Maude comments:

> The way society is now—so fast—everybody's touched. [She points to her head.] There's no time to know ourselves because there's so many things to do—a mother. At the hospital and EPIC there's time to think and get to know myself—why I am what I am. I have to learn to live with it. There's no cure for it. A fact is a fact. I don't like admitting I am a manic depressive, but you have to face facts.

Maude includes the burdens of motherhood in criticizing fast-paced modern society, which she sees as a contributor not only to her own personal problems but to those of people generally ("everybody's touched"). In so doing she offers a social explanation of her personal problems that bears some resemblance to the critical perspective outlined in Chapter 1. But no sooner spoken, this incipient critique is withdrawn in favor of the psychiatric disease model of the manic-depressive, which she then constructs as the central and permanent "fact" of her existence. This pattern brings to mind residents' initial attempts at social explanation and resistance to psychiatric authority in diagnostic interviews, only to be followed by acquiescence to psychiatric definitions.[2] What are the processes at work here? Maude again comments:

> I would go dancing for therapy [outside the hospital]. I don't dance with a partner, but get into my body and move—nothing really shocking—just dancing. In the hospital I was doing this, and some patients would join in. One staff got the doctor to observe and I stopped. I don't like just sitting around playing solitaire and listening to the radio. The psychiatrist asked me if I was getting messages from the radio, but I said I was just listening. [She laughs.]

Upon discharge from the hospital, Maude was able to obtain access to her patient records through the Freedom of Information Act. She found that she viewed her behavior in the hospital very differently than the staff did. What she saw simply as dancing was constructed in the staff notes as "symptoms of manic-depressive illness." More specifically, her performances were variously referred to in the following terms: "euphoric," "sexual preoccupation," "seductiveness," "psychotic gesturing," "posturing," "ritualistic behavior," and—"inappropriate."

Listening to the radio, which the psychiatrist questioned, was characterized in his notes as "internal preoccupation indicating probable hallucinations." Faced with the chronic boredom of institutional life, Maude says that she coped as best she could by dancing and listening to the radio (to the tune of amplified symptoms). And she claims that, though she stopped dancing under the doctor's scrutiny, as a result of her performance he prescribed an extra dose of drugs—which she was forced to take by injection after refusing to take them orally.

Like most residents, Maude admits that problems coping with everyday life led to her hospitalization. But she also says that her experiences while hospitalized and the ideas of staff strongly influenced her that the psychotic diagnosis of her situation was correct. She continues:

> I had a cousin who is manic depressive. She also had lots of kids to raise after her husband passed away. My brother after fighting Japan in World War II came back like that. He didn't want to kill anyone.

Maude again alludes to social dimensions plausibly implicated in her plight: Women like Maude and her cousin raising children in fatherless families (before the widespread development of support groups) and men like Maude's brother forced to kill against their wills. And from the diagnostic interviews we may recall Janice's story of caring for her family while still a child, and Efrem's soldiering and the synchronous tragic events at home.

The psychiatric explanation Maude has come to accept, however, has no room for the burdens of gender or other social constraints to constitute the psychic suffering of the person deemed mentally ill. On the contrary, all the individual's social and individual troubles now become the product of the illness. Accordingly, Maude squeezes the social accounts of troubles experienced by her cousin and brother, alongside her own, inside the explanatory grid of manic depression. (R) Eddie comments on an article EPIC staff gave him to help him understand his problems:

> It [the article, "Living with Schizophrenia"] showed me what I have. My wife is the stable one at home. She may divorce me. She has all the cards, it's her decision. I can't have a regular relation with my son because of my sickness. I'd like to stop putting myself down for my condition.

I ask Larry, the staff person who gave the article to Eddie, what he thinks the article's value is. Larry says that the article was written by a schizophrenic nurse who managed to get through training for this profession by paying careful attention to certain "rules of thumb" about the illness. Of chief value is the "sensible and straightforward" advice about taking "just the right amount of meds [psychiatric drugs] to control symptoms without snowing her so much she couldn't function." It provides the schizophrenic with important tips about diet and sleep, Larry adds, and talks about "early warning signs of the illness." In sum, it assumes that schizophrenia is a biochemical disease of the brain that is permanent and disabling to its sufferer, but that its symptoms can be somewhat controlled by careful attention to the coping strategies outlined.[3]

The article probably can help Eddie to stop blaming himself for his personal problems: he is "sick" and therefore not morally culpable or "bad." But it also teaches him, just as Maude was taught, to lay the entire conflict-ridden social world at the doorstep of a psychiatric disease category—in his case, schizophrenia. The article and other psychiatric ideological influences have the cumulative effect of predisposing residents to view their lives as appendages of their respective diseases. As such, these beliefs foreclose their ability to change problematic aspects of their social circumstances that may contribute to their unhappiness. (R) Maureen comments:

> It is an appalling state to have a psychiatrist decide I am psychotic. It is a shock to me. I'm angry and bitter. Is there no place I can go and live and be

in pain without having psychotic crap or pills, or orientation toward
self-destructive attitudes of psychologists and psychiatrists?

We recall that Maureen claims to communicate with people in heaven
(at least she did before taking psychiatric drugs). She also tells me that she
has psychic powers—specifically, visions of ordinary events about to
occur. Unlike Maude and Eddie, she vociferously rejects the psychiatric
construction of the complex mix of pain and wonder she bears. And like
Vern, she feels that psychiatric methods are subverting her spiritual
progress. But where can she go to "live and be in pain" without such
interference? (S) Clara comments:

> There were times people came through here [EPIC] who . . . said to people
> [staff], 'I'm not psychotic, I'm psychic.' And [staff] said, 'Huh, sure. We're
> gonna give you some meds, and we're not gonna validate that part of your
> experience. We're gonna look at the whole thing as psychosis.' And I think
> that's wrong. A lot of people could be considered psychotic because they
> have visions, hallucinations, and dreams, and use it as something positive.
> But if you already have a label on you . . . then people tend not to validate
> that side of your experience.

Clara in effect answers Maureen's desperate question. There is no place
to live without psychiatric interference while in this "unusual" state of
mind. She indicates that, at least at EPIC, the "master status" (Hughes
1945) of labeled psychosis drives out as illegitimate all competing social or
spiritual claims. Not only are psychic abilities rendered illegitimate, Clara
suggests, but emerging with the new psychotic tag is a new psychotic
identity to replace the resident's previous sense of self. And this new
identity gets reinforced by the forced ingestion of psychiatric drugs. Clara
thus validates residents' claims to this effect and other evidence we have
so far witnessed. (S) Kris, also a staff person, comments:

> Usually people are browbeaten by authority figures. They are given deep
> suggestions they are sick and must take them [drugs] or they will stay that
> way—or they just have to take them, period. There is no choice.

Kris both echoes and extends Clara's perspective. We have already
addressed the central place of drugs, but Kris links them more directly to
the process of labeling. According to Kris, staff's almost hypnotic "deep
suggestions" admonish residents ("browbeaten") that "they are sick,"
and further that they must take drugs or else stay sick for the rest of their
lives. By my count, 94 percent of residents, 290 of 309 who passed
through EPIC between 1981 and 1984, were put on psychiatric drugs.[4]
Very few, indeed, are permitted to "just say no."

Our culture believes that if a person requires drugs for any condition, whether physical or mental, this indicates that s/he is ill (Manning and Zucker 1976). Further, being considered ill carries with it the stigma of inferiority or contagion and implies but two remedies: complete cure or else quarantine, i.e., social exclusion. Thus residents are not only defined as ill, but are accordingly socially separated from the mainstream—by their very act of complying with staff's directives to take drugs in order not to be ill. Faced with this no-win situation, is it any wonder that most residents take leave of the drugs soon after leaving psychiatric settings? Condemned to illness and social exclusion both on and off drugs, most residents choose to live in this box while glimpsing the truth of their situation without side effects, that is, without drugs. (R) Simone comments:

> I have a strong feeling in the hospital and at EPIC that there's a conspiracy— and it's real. Staff keep writing and talking about me, but deny it. I may hear music that I'm not supposed to hear, but I'm not dense. I've lived too hard a life. I feel contained in a tube.

The psychiatric word for Simone's charge of "conspiracy" is "paranoia." But residents have reported that all aspects of their lives—physical, sexual, emotional, mental, and spiritual—are subject to staff's constant unsolicited probing and commentary. What's more, this commentary inevitably names them as mentally ill. Simone's perspective embraces these staff-alleged symptoms as the "music" she's "not supposed to hear", but belies staff's "therapeutic" model for them. She is intensely aware of the reality of her situation: corridors, locked rooms, video camera, staff notes, syringes—she feels "contained in a tube" with nowhere to hide. (R) Samuel comments:

> Psychotic means off the wall. It makes me feel worse than I am. It implies more trouble than most people, and there's nothing I can do about it. I've been diagnosed paranoid schizophrenic and manic-depressive. It's like calling me a dumb asshole, psycho, into drugs—really crazy. I don't get mad at people labeling me that way, but I'm uncomfortable. I don't know what it [psychotic] means except brain damaged. My problem is that I've been called so many things I start believing I'm psychotic because Doctor so-and-so said so. I don't want to believe that.

Nothing to Lose

Although, like Samuel, they "don't want to believe that," residents of psychiatric settings face an unavoidable public identity as mentally ill. (R) Shran comments:

Lots of people don't want anything to do with mental patients—including people's family and friends. My mother gets real uncomfortable with me, and talks to me like an illness—my sick Shran, my son the schizophrenic. When I went to the hospital I was living with roommates. When I got out they asked me to leave, which really upset me. I lost my job and most of my friends.

Shran indicates that, once his "master status" (Hughes 1945) as mentally ill became public, people (including family and friends) treated him as a cultural pariah. (R) Nanette comments:

'Manic depression' sounds like 'killer.' When people hear that they think you're really crazy, maybe violent, and they sometimes stay away.

Further, labeled psychotics like Shran and Nanette have been socialized in the same ways as "normals," notably through the educational system, the film industry, and electronic media (Nunnally 1961; Bissland and Munger 1985; Niedradzik and Cochrane 1985),[5] to learn what "everybody knows" about mentally ill people—namely, that they are dangerous, contagious, inferior, and worthy of social isolation. Thus the psychiatric judgment of people as mentally ill reinforces cultural stereotypes, which those so labeled then apply to themselves (Scheff 1984). In short, psychiatric prescriptions build upon and strengthen ordinary cultural programs for self-hate. (S) Cathy comments on (R) Erin's behavior:

Erin came to group [therapy] last night with dark glasses on, his hair slicked back, black boots, a black shirt with white piping on it, and white pants with a black stripe down the side. Then he stood up and called himself an insect! [Cathy laughs.]

Considered inferior and insignificant, Erin identifies himself as an insect (which, if it can elude the microscope, may scuttle from the blackness to sting his "betters"). This image both captures and satirizes his social circumstances. Erin's behavior suggests that a steady diet of bad news in psychiatric places often leads residents to grimace and pass it off with a smile. Forced smiles, jokes, and bravado become an umbrella for the deluge of embarrassments and humiliations residents encounter.

And these processes begin early on. The allegedly disruptive, odd, or otherwise misunderstood words and deeds of labeled-psychotic residents usually emerge within original families, are met initially by the disbelief, dismay, and consternation of family members, followed closely by the family's collusive and often desperate efforts to censure, redirect, or somehow "normalize" or contain such actions (cf. Goffman 1961, 1971; Spitzer and Denzin 1968). But typically the questionable behavior at some point spills into full public view, where it elicits police attention and, in short order, psychiatric intervention.[6]

Ironically, as we have seen, this intervention reproduces many of these original family patterns. Thus over time labeled psychotics begin to identify with, or even take a certain pride in, their membership in "Club Med." For example, a resident whose last name is Dixon and who for many years has been prescribed high doses of the psychiatric drug Prolixin, proudly calls himself "Prolixin Dixon." And there are other indicators of identification with this excluded/exclusive club. (R) Maude says:

> Wrap it up, I'm manic depressive, if you want to use the words. It's a commitment to living, it's never-never land.

Or as (R) Teresa puts it:

> I am psychoanalytically manic—or an open-minded and aware, creative person. I am only troubled by the depressive side.

And (R) Keenan boasts:

> I thought I was Christ—arms in the air, looking up into the sun, praising it. It took four cops to take me down and strap me up—that's a manic depressive, scary.

(R) Shran comments:

> Being crazy is like logrolling. You feel the excitement of trying to stay on top, and also the fear of falling at the same time. Trying to fit in with everybody else is like staying on the log. You know you can do it for a while, but sooner or later you must fall off. That's when you're different than everybody else and in your own world, and people don't want you around. You splash into the cold water.

Shran expresses the feeling that his life is out of his control, that "trying to fit in" with ordinary people will surely fail, just as one inevitably must fall off the log in the sport of logrolling. Residents of EPIC often present themselves in images suggesting that they see themselves as pawns of forces beyond their control or influence. And, as one learns soon, such images accurately express the location, status, and social experience of labeled psychotics as, in Shran's words, "different than everybody else," that is, as outsiders (Becker 1963). (R) Shran continues:

> Residents' topics of conversation 50 percent of the time is critical, negative, sarcastic, or as if we're victims. Other times they might talk about their

futures positively, or going somewhere to do something. But there's a support system to not do anything and lay back and that's considered funny and worthy of jokes.

Shran claims that among residents a pervasive outsider perspective "critical" of legitimate society prevails—a serious commitment to nonparticipation in legitimate society. Shran says that there is considerable mutual support to "lay back" as "victims." (R) Maude and (R) Keenan are talking:

Maude: Staff wants me to start looking for a job at the [sarcastic tone] "unemployment" department [California State Employment Service] tomorrow.
Keenan: That's "weept."
Maude: What does that mean?
Keenan: Weept. Broken-down, cracked, out of it, what's the use. There ain't no jobs for us there.
Maude: [Wearily,] Yeah.

This dialogue is typical of residents' conversations—especially when they are out of staff's earshot. We have documented that this seemingly cynical and pessimistic viewpoint is in fact rooted in residents' realistic assessment of their social illegitimacy. In lieu of other means of positive solidarity, residents come to identify with their record of failure in legitimate society. (R) Keenan comments:

I've seen the same people everywhere for years and years. I have an I.Q. of 134, but I can't understand why the same amount of people for so many years can't get cured. If they stay on [psychiatric] drugs, and some do, how come they can't perform and work? I'm just as bad. In 1974 I had a nervous breakdown. I worked 11 years at GE and then a breakdown, and never worked since. There isn't much sponging [on disability payments]. People are serious [about getting better]. One guy broke out, is doing fine working in a supermarket. The others are burnouts like vegetables—there's nothing else they can do.

Keenan begins by puzzling over why so few people escape his lot of labeled psychotic, but even before he finishes talking, he has gone far toward solving his own puzzle. Keenan despairs at seeing the "same people everywhere for years and years" not performing and working. We have seen that even those few who continue to take psychiatric drugs remain stuck in this no-win situation—locked in a box marked illness. And as witnessed in Keenan's conversation with Maude, labeled psychotics support one another's cynicism that society offers them no hope of success.

To see their reflections day after day, first in family abusiveness, and later in peers' gloomy faces and alibis for repeated failures, can only reinforce their self-construction in this light. While Keenan declares that "people are serious" about getting better, his scathing self- and subcultural portrait self-fulfillingly suggests that—for him and others like him—this has not been a possibility for a long time. Rather, he identifies himself as "just as bad" as his peers whom he also labels "burnouts like vegetables."

Not having worked for 11 years—a pattern typical of his peers— Keenan has nothing left to lose of legitimate society and only distant memories of its benefits. Unfortunately, were he not to continue communally identified with his psychotic subculture, which for him has become his trusted family, he would risk losing his only remaining concrete sources of personal succor and social solidarity.

In sum, residents like Shran, Maude, Teresa, Keenan, "Prolixin Dixon," and Erin come to identify with and even romanticize being cultural pariahs at the bottom of the social heap—from family to psychiatric suite. Having realized that they cannot win a claim to social legitimacy, many resign themselves to the role of illegitimate losers with little left to lose. Regrettably, they think and act accordingly.

This "tribal" commitment is not often so conscious or explicit, but like ivy grows subtly and diffusely—hardly noticed until one day it covers the house. No doubt for the most part labeled psychotics implicitly form unconscious and subliminal ties with the new ways. Rejected by legitimate society, they either accept the status of the losing underdog or feel the utter emptiness and isolation of a social vacuum—an intolerable condition for any human animal. (R) Maude comments:

> I've never been involved with the kind of people who are there [in the hospital and EPIC] before. Most people there feel like they were screwed as the weirdos of society. So we stopped playing dumb little games. Small things like not saying, 'please, can I have a cigarette,' just 'give me a cigarette.' There's less politeness and skills. If they [residents] asked you for a cigarette and you didn't give it to them, they might get real angry and blow up. They wouldn't cover it over like most people [outside the hospital]. There's a lot more direct feelings and thoughts, whether they're nice or nasty. I got more angry as a defense, and went off into fantasy things. . . . Nobody wants to talk about problems, there's a lot of silence. People are left to their own devices to work things out in that system.

People whose behavior is thought odd or disruptive by family and public alike typically meet kindred spirits for the first time in the hospital. As we have seen, after repeated stays in psychiatric settings—isolated from mainstream society amid failure and humiliation—many turn against its rituals and commitments. (In this regard, note the shift in Maude's own talk from *"they* were screwed as the weirdos of society" to, in the very next line, "so *we* stopped playing dumb little games.")

Maude suggests that hospitalized labeled psychotics become more direct and candid in expressing thoughts and feelings, jumping to the essentials in their discourse. Whether "nice or nasty," the polite veneer of everyday conversational ritual falls away. Maude also claims that she used anger "as a defense" against the starkly blunt talk. But in view of her remarks about candor, her increased anger may reflect the erosion of defenses—e.g., smiling when irritated—more than their maintenance.

In Maude's remarks is the implicit critique that legitimate society builds upon face-to-face deception. In fact, many critics have argued that defensive manipulation is the basis of public order, an idea also implicit in Goffman's (1959) concept of impression management. Or, as a recent TV commercial for deodorant put it, "Never let them see you sweat." As losers in our competitive society, labeled psychotics may have less motivation—rather than less ability—to maintain this deception. The general absence or decline of ritualistic politeness and other superficial gestures among them may occur because they have less or no reason to jockey for advancement, advantage, or otherwise enhanced social position.

Maude implicitly raises a fascinating related point. Maybe the permission labeled psychotics enjoy as social losers not to orient to others' expectations paradoxically provides more room to, as Maude puts it, go "off into fantasy things." As Maude indicates, when staff are not probing their behavior, labeled psychotics do not much talk spontaneously about mental or emotional "problems." And her comments about extensive "silence," with people "left to their own devices to work things out," suggest less selfishness and callous unconcern than tolerance for one another's idiosyncratic gestures. Without bothering to censure one another's often solipsistic bubbles of consciousness, they allow the internal psychic flow, fantasies and all, to spill into public view and earshot. In this sense there is not only more candor, but possibly a greater freedom in labeled-psychotic society than in legitimate society (without forgetting that reduced verbal production may also reflect painful self-preoccupation).

Perhaps it follows suit that people in psychiatric settings are more tolerant of brash, intrusive, or otherwise (by "normal" standards) disruptive and disarrayed activities. Again, residents for the most part provide mutual support for one another's fantastic tales or (mis)adventures, for "critical" and "negative" commentary on social conditions, and for "laying back" and thereby avoiding the ordinary everyday responsibilities—from cleaning one's room, making a shopping list, and buying groceries, to going to school or holding a job. After all, if one finds only futility in failed efforts to conform to legitimate society, as Keenan says, or repeatedly falls off the log, in Shran's image—then why not lick one another's wounds by making a virtue of the perceived necessity of failure? (R) Teresa comments:

> Psychiatrists want to control [in order] to function—especially time. When you get that [manically] high, you don't know what you're doing in terms of time. In manic highs there is no time—it's man-made—and everything flows together as it ought to be, the higher entities in control. There is perfect timing without the clock, but you can't work that way when you have a job and are living in society. Lots of people are robots. They don't think, are not open—robots. I don't want the mainstream, people who are afraid—people into pride, ego, vanity, lust, and greed.

Teresa critiques the control psychiatrists exercise as part of her larger critique of our time-bound culture, where technical means, e.g., the clock, and other tools, as Teresa suggests, become ends in themselves, which override moral values. Teresa also tells me that by "higher entities in control" she means intuitive and spiritual processes, which she sees as actively suppressed by the technical priorities built into our social organization. Her perspective resembles critical religious and political currents from both the Western and Eastern Worlds—from Marx and Weber to Christianity and Buddhism.

While Teresa is uncommonly articulate, her point of view reflects a central theme among labeled psychotics: a desire for a less pressured and even languid daily life in lieu of routinized activities, from household chores to jobs. As a consequence of their relegated status as "outsiders," labeled psychotics widely reject competitive egoism and conspicuous success, and their critique echoes the countercultural movement of the 1960s—or what (R) Samuel tersely summarizes as "trying to put job, school, life organized and blah, blah, blah." (R) Russell comments:

> I was living in a tent in the woods. For a long time I didn't clean it up, but then the necessity of insects, etc., and food, every coupla days I'd go downtown. . . . I thought I was taking pretty good care of myself—was getting exercise going back and forth to town. I was kicked back some, would sunbathe. I just didn't feel like I could really handle working.

Russell describes a life-style that, though perhaps shocking to middle-class sensibilities—we can imagine the "necessity of insects, etc."—he finds satisfactory (at least between hospitalizations). Russell suggests that he is more or less resigned to social circumstances like living in the woods and inability (or unwillingness) to work. By so doing he shifts the emphasis from the pain in the rite of passage to labeled-psychotic status, to the not altogether dark comfort in this role. Russell continues:

> If the system can't help and look out for me to get something going, then they shouldn't expect me to get any money or to pay them back. They shouldn't expect me to even, eh, to really do much, you know. I'm here because I have emotional and mental problems.

Russell declares that legitimate society should expect no contribution from him, since the "system" in his view did nothing to "help" or "look out" for him. There is implicit anger at his felt exclusion from jobs and so on ("get something going"). In effect, he says that since legitimate society made his bed for him, he will lie in it. If societal benefits have been denied him because of his "emotional and mental problems," he reasons, then by its own terms it cannot expect him to conform with its expectations as to life-style or anything else. Though Russell is resigned and even committed to his present outsider status, one senses his resentment.

Crazy Like a Fox

Many labeled psychotics, in solidarity with Russell's perspective, favor lackadaisical or perfunctory participation in psychiatric clinical activities. Labeled psychotics often go through the motions of attending group therapies, doing household chores, or performing outside volunteer work. But this activity is largely for staff's benefit, since residents wink at one another's erratic performances and almost invariably backslide into basic nonparticipation at the earliest opportunity—often after an ostensibly successful stay in the psychiatric setting. Again, in (R) Russell's words:

> Cathy [staff] said Christmas is over, you haven't found housing or tried yet, you're gonna have to leave. I felt that was cold. I just really felt upset, and sometimes when I get upset the idea of suicide comes in there. I have hardships and stuff and then I feel a little bit more than others, and things get pretty heavy. I just thought I had a few more days, that I could start preparing myself. I was starting preparing myself anyway. Christmas is what messed it up, or made it a little bit different.

During the colder times of year Russell seeks shelter in psychiatric settings. But the hospital and EPIC provide far more than just literal shelter, for, as we have seen, they are "home" to the labeled-psychotic tribe—perhaps most significantly at Christmas. And if push comes to shove, Russell is ready to use his threat of suicide to lever psychiatric staff into allowing him to stay.

Every psychiatric hospital crisis or intake staff person knows that this suicide gambit is the major ploy by which labeled psychotics (and others) get off the streets and out of the cold. Russell calls (S) Cathy "cold" for asking him to leave EPIC after Christmas is over, and by so doing intends (though it may be more unconscious than that) to hook her guilt in order to wheedle continued housing and/or emotional support. The implicit message is that if the spurned resident were to kill him/herself, the staff person would be to blame.

And the strategy often works—especially if there is any evidence of suicide attempts in the past. Although these gestures usually fall far short of success (the most common being superificial wrist cuts or knowingly nonlethal drug overdoses), the staff person must treat both threats and simulated attempts seriously. Not to do so could cast doubt on the staff person's emotional and professional fitness—especially if the rejected person were actually to commit suicide. Every staff person has heard stories of these occurrences. Thus psychiatric staff most often err on the conservative side. The suicidal claimant usually gains entry to the hospital.

There is another way labeled psychotics "break into" the hospital (if the door is locked from the wrong side). (R) Erin comments:

> I was walking down the street talking and tripping to myself. I guess I got kind of loud, because a cop walked up to me. I told him I needed protection. I admitted to being part of two murders. I had no direct involvement, but felt I was part of them. The cop took me to the hospital. The murders were in the paper. He took me here [to the hospital] because I can't be responsible.

By presenting himself publicly as delusional and out of control, Erin thoroughly plays the stereotypical psychotic. After Erin is brought to the hospital by the police, psychiatric staff tend to view his behavior as conservatively as they do suicidal claims. Namely, if the guy is "really crazy," i.e., gravely disabled in some sense, he should be off the streets. Since the police, psychiatric staff, and the rest of us are not God, we cannot be sure just how "responsible"—how "out of control"—Erin really is, or is able to be. By posing as a disruption to public order—and adding tales of remote psychic direction of murder and other unusual beliefs—he obtains a sure ticket to the hospital. Crazy like a fox, Erin comes home.

We have gone from addressing the initial desperation residents often feel in diagnostic interviews to exploring their gradual personal and subcultural identification with labeled-psychotic status. As we have seen, whether darkly or humorously resigned to their plight or manipulating what few benefits remain to be had, labeled psychotics ironically come to identify with their ill-starred psychological, cultural, and economic status at least as thoroughly as psychiatric staff ascribe it to them.

A simple analogy may help to summarize and clarify the distinctions we have addressed in the transition from normal to labeled psychotic. Having been forced to wear ill-fitting shoes, labeled-psychotics' feet at first pinch, then cut, and burn unbearably. But in time their feet go numb, and finally, they hardly feel the pain. The erstwhile poorly fitting shoes now in a sense "fit"—or at least the numbness makes them less troublesome. In any case, with no new shoes in sight, labeled psychotics learn to make a virtue of necessity.

Closing this "psychotic circle," as it were, the people of this tribe can, ironically, only retain some sense of human viability by embracing their social illegitimacy as outsiders. But this circle is part of a still larger circle, which (R) Shran characterized as the "patienthood/staffhood syndrome." We turn now to address the psychiatric staff of EPIC—or the psychiatric "border patrol."

Notes

1. Phenothiazines are the major culprit. Lithium is not implicated in this condition, but nonetheless is a very dangerous drug. Besides the effects Maureen mentions below (plus sweating and muscle weakness in some, and great thirst in most people), it can damage kidneys, and blood concentrations in relatively small amounts can cause death. The conservative *Physician's Desk Reference*, its information on drug side effects provided by the drug companies (and readily available to staff in most psychiatric facilities), opens the blurb on lithium with a boldface warning: "Warning:" Lithium toxicity is closely related to serum Lithium levels, and can occur at doses close to therapeutic levels. "Facilities for prompt and accurate serum Lithium determinations should be available before initiating therapy" (Physicians Desk Reference 13XX:1789).

2. Since this was an early interview in my study, it has occurred to me that Maude may have begun critically, but then fearfully projected me as a psychiatrist and told me what she thought I wanted to hear.

3. See especially Sarbin and Mancuso (1980) and Abrams and Taylor (1983). Both studies survey and analyze the schizophrenia literature, with Abrams and Taylor focusing on the alleged genetic evidence. The authors of both studies maintain that the concept confuses the empirical processes in this human suffering. In short, they contend that there is little or no evidence that schizophrenia exists as a disease entity.

4. This figure includes residents on routine and "PRN" (i.e., ad hoc, occasional) regimens of lithium, phenothiazines, phenothiazinelike, and miscellaneous antidepressant drugs.

5. Although the Nunally (1961) study is almost thirty years old, its chief finding that the mass media promote stereotypes of "psychotics" has dramatically deepened with the enormous expansion of the culture industry and its sensational products, e.g., from *Psycho* to the seemingly endless *Friday the 13th* series of

films. The studies by Bissland and Munger (1985) and Niedradzik and Cochrane (1985) explore this issue in the more contemporary social context.

6.   My interviewees report essentially similar patterns of family reaction to their behavior, i.e., collusive action by family, police, psychiatric authorities, and so forth, as found by Goffman (1961:127–69) and Denzin and Spitzer (1966:265–71).

Chapter 3

BORDER PATROL

> Being mental health workers fits who they are: fringe people working with other fringe people (Kris, psychiatric staff).

As we go about our daily lives, we hope our performances will earn for us the rewards promised by our audiences—especially those closest and most significant to us like family, friends, lovers, or bosses. Meanwhile, "backstage" our mental life is probably in a lot more disarray than we typically let on in public. We are often not as sure of what we are doing and why we are doing it as we would like other people to believe. The same is true, of course, for psychiatric staff. In this chapter we will explore motivations prominently involved in staff's patrolling the murky psychic waters between "sanity" and "insanity."

Psychiatric Boot Camp

When talking about their personal lives, EPIC staff frequently bring up their family backgrounds. Further, they often connect these origins with present emotional orientations toward their lives:

Susan: I'm too concerned with others. I played the counselor role in our family when my mom and brothers conflicted, and both talked to me about it. . . . My mom was an alcoholic. . . . I'm still too shy and passive in asserting my needs.

Kris: I've basically developed in isolation. My parents weren't there when I needed them. Basically I spent a lot of time at home, sick a lot—like a little prison. . . . I see myself as a person in conflict. I always have a kind of thorn in my side. I put lots of attention into trying to get it out.

51

There's always something happening here. [He looks down at his side and tugs at it.] I've lived my life that way.

Brenda: I'm giving away power in my own relations, but coming across as autonomous. It's an old pattern. As a child in my family I hid my feelings to take care of my family and was very sad.

Lela: I'll cover up my insecurities. I strive to carry myself with self-confidence, but I don't feel it.

Brad: When I feel really bad, I feel pressure in my chest. I feel like I will explode with pressure and tension. That happens because of relationships. . . . It's cyclic. Sometimes I notice lability, mood swings.

Nadine: I tend to get paranoid. I tend to get out of perspective a lot. I drive myself nuts. . . . I was hospitalized in 1970 for 18 months. . . . My negative qualities outweigh the positive. I'm obsessive and have very high, unforgiving expectations of everybody and myself. People get bent out of shape by that.

Most of the original families of EPIC staff are rife with emotional turmoil, including conflict, alcoholism, and neglect. Insecurity about personal and social competence is also a dominant theme, as is the strategy of masking emotional pain with a show of public strength. In Lela's words, "I'll cover up my insecurities. I strive to carry myself with self-confidence, but I don't feel it." (Staff's use of psychiatric terms like "lability," "mood swings," "paranoid," and "obsessive" to describe their troubles reflects phenomena I call "closet insanity" and "reverse role modeling," which we will explore fully later.)

How is this compensatory interpersonal strategy learned? As exemplified in Brenda's and Susan's accounts, most staff indicate that they had roles as caretakers or peacemakers in their families. Three report that they took care of alcoholic parents; two said they nurtured labeled-psychotic parents. In fact, 86 percent of staff (24 of 28) see themselves as having been de facto counselors—embattled referees in families shot through with sadness, anger, and addiction. And hiding feelings in order to take care of adult family members was a central role requirement, which staff learned and identified with early on. Further, a majority are conscious that their present work roles reprise these early performances. They have become paid professional caretakers based upon the childhood model that dictated that their own needs would be indirectly met by helping others.

Staff report that the biggest problem in their present lives is still that they do not take adequate care of their own personal needs. As Susan puts it:

It's important for staff to take care of our needs enough that we can emotionally take care of clients. We don't do as well as we could. We go home and get into drugs and alcohol.

Maybe because of their socialization for martyrdom as family caretakers, professional caretakers sometimes, as in Nadine's case, collapse under the burden and become objects of care themselves. While Nadine is one of only two staff members who alluded to a history of mental hsopitalization, I suspect there are others. However, as we learned in Chapter 2, such an admission opens one up to the social stigma and exclusion attendant to labeled mental illness. And nobody knows that better than psychiatric staff.

Camaraderie of Misfits

We have seen that staff are launched into the world from quite thorny nests, and most also find the world a quite difficult place. For example, while the majority have not experienced much trouble with schooling,[1] most admit to spotty and erratic work records. After much aimless meandering about in their careers, however, staff finally came home to roost as beleaguered caretakers—this time for the featherless birds of society instead of their own families. (S) Cathy depicts her odyssey:

> I bounced around in a lot of marginal, shitty, "studenty" jobs—waitressing and stuff. [Then] I stumbled into mental health through serendipity, having a lover who was a psych graduate student. Our two best friends were also psych grad students and we all moved here. I was immersed every night, sitting around the dinner table, and I said, 'This sounds like real interesting stuff.' I was unemployed, there was an ad in the paper for a job in a mental hospital, and I got the job. As a kid I wanted to be a surgeon, but I took the escape route.

Cathy is typical of psychiatric workers in that she "stumbled into" this career. Cathy is atypical, however, in that her early ambition to become a doctor was at least consistent with her eventual "escape route" into the less rigorous and prestigious but more accessible psychiatric work. At least the manifest purpose of both jobs is to lessen human pain. (S) Melissa gives this account of her entry into this work:

> I came to Lakeside and was unemployed—I took anything. It was an accident. I started at the laundry in the hospital and it looked like they [psychiatric staff] were having a lot of fun. I asked to be a psych aide, and fell into it.

For Melissa there is no sense of related early purpose, only serendipity. Similarly, Lance, the supervisor of EPIC, says even he got "sucked into" psychiatric work. And he adds that he thinks most staff similarly "stumble into mental health after they've done a lot of things," that they are "thrust into mental health and just latch onto it." His viewpoint is typical of staff. As (S) Kris comments:

> It's [psychiatric work] like a vacuum. If you don't have a tight grasp on other things, it sucks you into it. There's a certain 'pulling effect.' If you don't want to be an executive or haven't found another niche.

Many of the images running through staff accounts (e.g., "fell into," "sucked into") similarly suggest surrender to forces beyond control. No staff gave me a sense of inspired calling for psychiatric work. In fact, I experienced staff as often running from what they disliked rather than toward what they felt they must do. As Ken says, "I was in engineering and was dissatisfied with that. . . . Psych(ology) was one of the more interesting areas. I did well in it." While most staff express some fondness for their unintentional careers, the impression nonetheless remains that the person finally found something s/he could do successfully after many false starts and failures. Kris elaborates upon his perception of staff's background motives for entering the field:

> It's their own confusion in their life, past, present, future—working out their own confusion with other people. . . . Some people are drifters and just fall into it like flypaper. . . . It's a place for insecure people to come and stay in. There's a security found in no other jobs out there, and people not good at very much else in a tangible way.

Thus it appears that for many staff the initial choice of psychiatric career is more a default amid personal confusion and insecurity than a clear or conscious choice. Besides a general lack of other marketable skills, virtually all staff admit that some form of emotional dissonance figured into their choice of careers, and that psychiatric work seemed to provide indirect help. In (S) Ken's words, "I had enough personal problems to question myself—what I was about and what made other people tick." And in light of the caretaking role so prominent in staff biographies, the need to know how oneself and others "tick" probably includes the (perhaps unconscious) compulsive need to be needed.

Lest I be too hard on staff, I suspect this pattern is not unlike the combination of ordinary obligations and serendipity that locks other workers into their jobs. As in any other line of work, no doubt many staff remain in this field out of practical inertia, having built up a psychiatric job resume over the years as what they "do." Further, many studies of work have shown that workers in all careers (including unpaid "home-makers") are conflict-ridden, insecure, confused, even terrorized (Rubin 1976; Sennett and Cobb 1973; Terkel 1975).

In view of this, one may interpret Kris' words, "There's a security found in no other jobs out there," as an intelligent response to a limited and limiting job market. For one thing, relatively candid communication in psychiatric settings stands in marked contrast to a more censored interaction in most other public places (Goffman 1959:67,71). In a sense, just as the psychiatric setting offers a home to residents, it also offers the feeling of home to staff. Emotional pain is often permitted a public airing amid considerable empathy, and public talk generally is often playful, freewheeling, and humorous.

Why is this so? No doubt part of the answer lies in the fact that psychiatric work, as ideological work, is not under the direct gun of efficient labor disciplines required in production or even sales work. Without a concrete product or service to produce for exchange, staff have less pressure to be "on center stage" and have, as a corollary, more permission to let their hair down in this "backstage" occupation. This sanctuary is no small benefit of psychiatric work.

While staff may enjoy asylum from having to adjust to the overarching alienation of mainstream workplaces, they also feel a certain disconnectedness. The institutional location of psychiatric work as a "borderland" outside the ken of central productive industries may serve to reinforce staff's identification with social–psychological marginality as sketched so far. Let us consider the following excerpts:

Clara: It's just how the world is today. We [staff] look around and see everything messed up and in a state of chaos, all the hatred and violence. . . . People are judged by their appearance. As a minority I'm judged for my appearance too. [She is obese.] And there's really assholes out there who are blatantly nasty for no reason.

Nadine: Life is all a passing show, a game. I used to get lost in tragic emotion with a horrible ending. Now I try not to get attached to any of it. Life is all bullshit.

Kay: Most people who are normal achievers are petrified of breaking through and letting down control to discover what's out there. I'm afraid too, but I'm more afraid of not finding out what's beyond this dusty level. Life has given me material things that are supposed to make it for you—but I'm dissatisfied.

Cathy: I always was an intellectual—at least I wanted to be. I wanted to have that as my image. I got . . . . a sense of how rejected that was, and it was important to me.

Jim: What it relates to is frustration in terms of conflict as I move through the social world and deal with all the stuff I have to do and cope with it. . . . I have tremendous concerns about a lot of the ethics and values promulgated by the current form of corporate capitalism—it's incredibly destructive.

Nigel: I feel disgust for questions of normality. I don't live by 'normal'
             criteria. At times I feel abnormal in this society. There are parts of me
             that have had to readjust.

This portrait shows staff looking askance at life as, among other things,
a "passing show" of "bullshit." In fact, every staff person interviewed
harbors some disgruntled dislike for major aspects of everyday life as they
experience it—often termed "the system." Many also report that "mainstream" society often returns the favor by reacting with xenophobia to
their personal physical and cultural differences: As examples, staff claim
to be the target of homophobia (Nigel is gay), anti-intellectualism (Cathy),
antifat narcissism (Clara), and antireligious and political radicalism (Kay
and Jim). Thus staff, who are fraught with personal insecurities and drift
into this work in tandem with default in straight jobs, also object to
dominant cultural realities, toward which they feel marginal. In short,
staff share a common subcultural identification as outsiders (Becker
1963). In Kris' words:

> Unskilled people get into mental health work. . . . It's people who are
> drifting, unless they are professional psychology students; sometimes
> intellectuals; sometimes happy-go-lucky people; sometimes sociopaths
> [note: manipulators]—but they don't fit into the mainstream well. A
> struggling musician had nothing tangible enough, so plugged into mental
> health. It's a camaraderie of misfits. With me, I was in this counterculture
> thing and said, 'What's this mental health about?'

Kris' question is in fact the occasion of this study: "What's this mental
health about?" While my subsequent text will attempt to answer this
question fully, the shorthand version can be stated now: Psychiatric work
is mostly about the "mental health" of the staff. We turn now to explore
these processes.

                                Closet Insanity

Staff are enabled to build the wall marking the border between "sanity"
and "insanity," thereby establishing the psychiatric enterprise, by means
of a peculiarly problematic relationship with the residents—a relationship
that will be at the center of our subsequent investigation. The following
excerpts are from staff accounts of their "unusual experiences."

Nadine: I'm against psychiatric drugs from personal experience. I'm more
              qualified here. I've been on both sides of the fence. I don't know if I
              should talk about this. [I assure her that all information will be totally

confidential.] I was hospitalized in 1970 for 18 months, and on and off for three years have been on Stelazine, Thorazine, Imipramine, Valium, Librium, for several years. [Her list includes both major "antipsychotic" tranquilizers and minor tranquilizers]. I could have become a prescription drug addict. I'm not ashamed of the experience, but people in the mental health profession stigmatize.

Nadine offers "both sides of the fence" as her personal reality. She hastens to add: "I don't know if I should talk about this." Reassured, she goes on to reveal her prolonged mental hospitalization and dependency on major psychiatric drugs. Her candor notwithstanding, Nadine is fearful about having publicly disclosed this history. Although I defined my status as a "neutral" sociological researcher to each staff person and resident,[2] Nadine knows that as a psychiatric worker she would be likely to define *her own* background as continuing evidence of psychosis (at least "in remission"). As she puts it, "people in the mental health profession stigmatize."

Karla: I see myself as a witch and pagan. I do rituals and ceremonies like that—and altered states of psychic ability. I'm real cautious about revealing unusual states, because I have no experience to justify them to peers. . . . I can more or less do "out of body" experiences at will. I've had memories of previous lives. I know I lived in the time of the persecution of witches, and that I died twice. I'm really uptight about telling you this. I don't express this to people at work. I know it's confidential, but I'm afraid. [I reassure her.] There is prejudice against calling oneself witches—satanic, devil-worshipping, etc. There's a stigma.

Karla recognizes that her tale of witchery, unusual psychic states, past lives, and the like put her in danger within a psychiatric context of meaning. She knows further that all claims without ready empirical corroboration are the stuff she herself as a psychiatric worker labels psychotic delusion. That is why, right after this public admission, she virtually panics, saying she is "uptight" and "afraid" about revealing these experiences "to people at work."

Clara: A disembodied arm with a knife stalked me in the hall of my parents' home. I sometimes hear voices in the wind calling my name. At 16 a spirit—I think of my dead grandmother—picked me up and dropped me on my bed. That's why I'm asking, is this confidential? [She laughs nervously.] Certain people you don't tell these kinds of things to, like my mother said when I was young. I wouldn't feel anywhere near as

comfortable talking with you if I hadn't known you from before. Some
of this stuff, if I had told a psychiatrist, they'd throw away the key.

Similar to Karla, Clara's story of otherworldly and other unusual
psychic phenomena gives her fearful pause about how confidential these
admissions are. Like Karla, she realizes that such revelations within a
psychiatric frame of reference lead to a psychotic diagnosis. As she puts
it, "if I had told a psychiatrist, they'd throw away the key."

> *Sidney:* I have real crazy thoughts sometimes, but the catch is I don't act on
> those kinds of things. [I ask him to describe what he calls "crazy
> thoughts."] Sorry, those thoughts are *mine.* [Strong emphasis.]

Although he alludes to thoughts he calls "crazy," Sidney refuses to give
them any specific content. His response departs from typical staff
reactions as depicted above. However, Sidney's emphatic insistence on
keeping these thoughts private suggests that he shares his fellow staff's
fears that public disclosure of their content might elicit a diagnosis of
mental illness.

> *Lela:* In the ninth grade I felt I had a schizophrenic break for a short time. I
> heard voices and felt a strange paranoia all the time. I was lethargic, more
> than my usual laziness. I was very depressed, slightly suicidal, misera-
> ble. The voices were flat, the words unintelligible. I heard my name
> called. A few of the words they said I heard in my head repeatedly. They
> were very familiar, though they were unintelligible. But I couldn't grasp
> them and repeat them to people. I felt real dead and blank. I had a flat
> affect when I talked. I was seeing a psychiatrist at the time, but I never
> told him. I was afraid he would lock me up. Schizophrenia may be a
> matter of admission or denial. A "schizophrenic" is someone who
> admits going through experiences like mine. If I did get labeled schizo-
> phrenic then, it would be hard to shake off the label. I could be
> institutionalized now.

Lela's revelation of her unusual experiences is untypical of staff in that
she shows no fear or ambivalence about these disclosures (at least not
outwardly). When first exposed to psychiatry as a youth, however, she
was not so dauntless. On the contrary, she fearfully attempted to conceal
these experiences, and by so doing demonstrated a precocious savvy
about the power of labeling. As she puts it, "If I did get labeled
schizophrenic then, it would be hard to shake off the label. I could be
institutionalized now."

Lela unabashedly uses terms like "schizophrenic break," "paranoia,"
and "flat affect" to define her experiences within the conceptual framework of labeled psychosis. By so doing, Lela manifests what I introduced

earlier as "reverse role modeling," which includes staff's use of psychiatric criteria to define or describe their own personal difficulties. While reverse role modeling is typical of staff, most also take pains publicly to mask or rationalize private fears that their own difficult or odd behavior indicates mental illness. I call this paradoxical twin phenomenon of reverse role modeling "closet insanity."

Similar to Lela's youthful trepidation, most staff are ambivalent about revealing their unusual experiences to me. They have difficulty deciding whether to take me as sociological researcher as promised, or psychiatric diagnostician as feared.

What is the source of this wary ambiguity? Staff spend many hours in the company of people labeled psychotic. Staff's frequent contact tends to increase their (largely unconscious) emulation of the residents' gestures and identification with their status—the essential meaning of reverse role modeling. Through this intimate daily association, staff come to see that many of their own unusual experiences, while hidden from public view or "in the closet," mirror those of the residents. Through both conscious and unconscious reverse role modeling and staff's fear of being labeled (closet insanity), they project a kind of "reverse diagnostic interview" onto my interview context. As such, they evaluate their own experiences through the ideology of psychosis by which they understand the daily behavior of the residents and which, in accordance with their indoctrination in positivist psychiatry, they believe is objective.

Since "out of body" and other unusual psychic experiences are identical for staff and residents, staff fear that their identities may be interchangeable—that they may be or may become "objectively" psychotic by their own yardstick. In Clara's words, "Certain people [i.e., psychiatrists and other staff] you don't tell these kinds of things too. . . ." As a reaction against her (largely unconscious) reverse role modeling and feared closet insanity, Clara responds in the context of our interview—which I explicitly defined as open-ended—as if she were a labeled psychotic telling her symptoms to a psychiatrist. Accordingly, she both fears and expects that I (he) will diagnose her as insane.

Patrolling the Border

People who want to work in mental health are drawn to it. It implies you are doing good in the world and are a "together person." In reality you don't have to be together to help others. I'm being tongue-in-cheek, but it's true (Karla).

We have seen that staff experience what they suspect to be closet insanity. We now turn to explore the conceptual ways staff attempt to ward off this threat by distinguishing both their thoughtways and behavior from those of the residents, i.e., how staff attempt to convince themselves and everybody else that they are on the right side of the wall after all. (In Chapter 4 we will examine the behavioral ways staff distinguish themselves from residents as part of their work activity.)

Staff contrast themselves with labeled psychotics in four basic, interrelated ways:

1. Staff contend that they cope better with emotional pain and everyday problems.
2. Staff claim that they have both less and less severe private problematic experiences.
3. Staff hold that their unusual experiences are more real.
4. Staff claim that their biology is more normal.

These dimensions will be illustrated by the following excerpts from staff accounts of their unusual experiences and my subsequent commentary:

On Coping

>   *Craig:* The pain they [the residents] have to get away from may be like my pain and different. The intensity for them may be a little sharper, more acute—but it's still pain. But my way and their way of dealing with it is different. They want to go out and have a good time too: fuck off, have a drink, be with friends, be by themselves. They do what they do, I do what I do. I don't think we do it a whole lot different. . . . How I live with it—the amount of time I'm away from pain, or that I'm not directly in touch with it, or can ignore it, or somehow avoid it—that's the difference: My avoiding techniques work a little bit better in this world than their avoiding techniques do.

Craig admits that he suffers emotionally just as residents do. However, he claims that he does so less intensely because of better "avoiding techniques" for coping with his emotional pain. However, my attempts to elicit the specific ways in which he thinks his methods of avoidance are "different" and "better" than those of residents come up empty. He offers no content for this contrast. On the contrary, he outlines identical ways in which staff and residents avoid their pain (e.g., drinks and being with friends) and thus curiously undermines his position. One concludes that the truth of Craig's claim is less important than its strategic ideological function to create social–psychological distance between his and the residents' psychological suffering.

>   *Clara:* I look around and see everything messed up and in a state of chaos. Residents choose to hibernate, and detach themselves, but I try to methodically, step-by-step, plug through. Our thinking is a lot clearer,

where they get so jumbled from so much stimulation. It seems we can sort things out a little easier: This is what we need to do to get from here to there, and compartmentalize, rather than being so overwhelmed by everything.

We have a different overall outlook. Life may be messed up and going wrong—your experience is valid, but where will you go from here? That's the difference. Staff can plug through everyday stuff and live the bare bones of their life as best they can, and find the pleasures here and there. Residents just pull the blankets over their heads. I have questions about how much control these people just give away. [I ask her whether she means that residents let their problems take over their world, while staff do not.]

Yes, to some degree. The question is, how much of your control . . . choice are you going to throw away? How strong are you going to be to shape what's going on? How much are you able to compartmentalize or detach yourself from what's going on . . . able to say, "I know all this is happening, but what can I do with my life?"

Clara claims that staff sympathize with the difficulty labeled psychotics encounter in trying to cope with the "messed up" modern world. She thus reveals staff's outsider cultural orientation discussed earlier. She also holds that labeled psychotics cannot think as clearly as staff because they are overwhelmed by "stimulation" (the source and character of which are left unexamined.) The upshot of this alleged difference is that staff are better able to cope with terrible modern life.

However, Clara's sympathetic identification with residents' outsider status and her explanation for their woes in terms of "jumbled" thinking only go so far. Clara's protest that residents are better able to function in everyday life than they let on also show staff's frustrated weariness from the hard work of attempting to motivate them. She in effect complains that residents' withdrawal from everyday responsibilities is at least in part a willful default on their ability to cope. When she remarks, "How much are you able to compartmentalize or detach yourself from what's going on?" we may detect her resentment of having to work so hard to mask her own emotional pain in order to cope with this rough-and-tumble world. Clara essentially puts forth a "bootstrap" ideology of rugged individualism: If staff must suppress their own considerable psychological suffering in order to face daily demands, why can't—or better, why don't the residents? This distinction implicitly introduces a claim for staff's moral superiority, and veers close to blaming the victims for their plight.

On Severity

Lela: Residents and staff are similar in that we all are human and have problems, but some have more than others. Nobody's life is without difficulties. Staff tend to have higher education, better job skills, better social skills, more effective strategies for dealing with the world. I suspect that a lot of staff have had, if they are not ex-patients, some experiences in life which have been something like residents have experienced, from alcoholism to breakdowns. A lot have had heavy problems in the past, but learned more effective coping mechanisms.

Lela suggests that staff's and residents' problems in living differ more in number and severity than in kind. Claiming that the lives of both groups have been fraught with psychological pain (to which this research attests) she also alleges, like all staff, that the border between both groups consists of staff's "more effective" coping mechanisms. And she specifies education and social and job skills as key variables in this construction. (In Chapter 4 we will see how psychiatric "job skills" fit into this picture.)

> *Lorelei:* My father was hospitalized as a schizophrenic and manic-depressive. So was my mom—but she functions. I was programmed very nicely in my family to be a scapegoat. I had a general lack of family and friends and knowing how to take care of myself. But there's a distinction between being "chronic" and just once, like myself. One crisis person may not come back, but "chronics" haven't learned proper support, balance.

Lorelei is among the staff who were caretakers of labeled-psychotic parents. And her "scapegoat" self-definition relative to her original family suggests that she may have martyred herself on behalf of her family, a pattern typical of staff as discussed above. Lorelei labels herself as a "crisis person" whose problems in living are less severe than "being chronic." In the parlance of psychiatric ideology, the word "chronic" is a euphemism for a long-term, hopeless career labeled psychotic, whereas "crisis" connotes a one-time-only brush with psychotic labeling.

Lorelei attributes chronics' inability to recover to their failure to learn how to gain "proper support, balance." Thus she insinuates that even staff with some psychiatric history who achieve this state, like herself, enjoy a superiority to labeled psychotics who do not—a claim reminiscent of Carla's view that labeled psychotics willfully default on their ability to cope. Our examination of the sources of staff's allegedly greater support and balance in Chapter 4, however, may lead to a different conclusion.

On Reality

> *Susan:* When I'm tired, I have optical illusions—whatever you call them. I misinterpret gestures or movements. I see things that are not there, but

it's more of a play on light than fantasy or delusions like our clients. My experiences are when I'm overly tired or drug induced. I think residents really believe that it's there—really see it and hear it. I do think there are chemical differences between us and them.

Susan claims that her unusual experiences include mistaking visual or auditory events for reality when they are not occurring. She implies that she temporarily believes such observations to be real, only to discover their unreality later. As to what makes her "misinterpret" these phenomena, she offers lighting conditions, fatigue, and drugs as situational causal explanations. Conversely, she claims that labeled psychotics believe in the reality of such mistaken observations, and appears to suggest that they persist in such beliefs despite contrary evidence—are, in a word, deluded.

All staff similarly contrast their alleged ability to distinguish reality from unreality with its alleged absence in labeled psychotics. Further, all staff provide some rational (usually biological) causal explanation for this difference, intended to prove that they are objectively sane, while residents are objectively insane. As Susan put it, "there are chemical differences between *us* and *them*" [my emphasis].

Joan: I receive thoughts which are a gift from outside me, rather than from my own consciousness. There's a sensation of energy moving through my body, a physical sensation, and extending out of my body, particularly my hands. I feel like I receive guidance on personal questions from a higher source: simply, open surrender to whatever happens, to God. I ask God what it's like to get "yes," and ask what happens. Then I ask what it's like to get "no." The goal is the unconscious source of information—God. . . .

When self-esteem is nonexistent, like with many residents, then there is crisis enough to give the unconscious messages to take over. It throws up information and tells the resident it's real. It's a projection of unconscious imagery, but residents believe it's real. At least they interact with that material as if it were outside themselves. It's the separation from its emotional content—sadness, anger, fear, and their nonrecognition—which results in schizophrenic behavior.

Joan claims that she receives personal advice from God in a directly physical way. She defines herself elsewhere as a "transpersonal psychologist," and says she believes that God is the unconscious source or life force behind all manifest realities in the world. Her view is that one ought always to use one's conscious mind in the quest to tap into one's unconscious—a direct aspect of God. As she puts it here, "The goal is the unconscious source of information—God."

While Joan sketches a positive view of the unconscious relative to her unusual experiences, she characterizes the unconscious of residents negatively. This contrast hinges on her claim that residents lack self-esteem (a claim just as plausibly applicable to staff). In any case, Joan claims that her unconscious is the bearer of ultimate reality or God, and conversely, that residents' unconscious is the bearer of ultimate unreality as "projection" and "schizophrenic behavior."

On Normality

> *Lorelei:* Psychologically and physically there's something deficient causing the problem of their faulty reality testing. It's like epilepsy. Most of these residents have a thought disorder caused by an imbalance in their chemical system which makes them very susceptible to stress. It's a biological and inherited problem.

Lorelei claims that defective biology underlies both the alleged inability of labeled-psychotic residents to perceive reality correctly and their vulnerability to "stress." Likening psychosis to the brain disorder epilepsy, she contends that residents suffer from a chemically induced "thought disorder" with a genetic ("inherited") cause.

> *Kris:* Residents putting blood on themselves, tying three knots in an undershirt because it's a magic formula: Something in them *is* abnormal physiologically. Something in them is making them very different than others: a different biology, different stimuli, and thus different responses.

Kris claims that the ritualistic actions of labeled-psychotic residents, part of "a magic formula," are caused by something abnormal "physiologically," excluding all social explanations, "something *in them*" (my emphasis). In good positivist fashion, he contends that their "different biology" generates "different stimuli," which produce "different responses" in a neatly linear causal chain of command.

We're All the Same, But . . .

Remember that while Craig and Clara claim that they cope with psychological pain and the demands of everyday life better than residents do, they also know implicitly that this capacity depends on the continuation of the status quo. They are therefore haunted by the question, Will it always be so? After all, staff spend most of their waking hours with people who overtly enact the psychic pain that they—with "coping mechanism helmets" strapped in place—also covertly experience. Staff must actively suppress or redirect the identical feelings and feelings of identification with residents in order to do their job. The key (largely unconscious) danger of reverse role modeling is that staff's closet insanity always threatens to overwhelm their strategic defenses—and burst into full public view.

It is instructive to look at the account of our aforementioned transpersonal psychologist, Joan. We recall that she applies her psychoanalytically derived model to very similar psychic phenomena in two mutually exclusive ways: negatively to residents' "false" reality, and positively to her "true" reality. But how does Joan *know* that her unconscious embodies God or life force as reality, while the unconscious of the labeled-psychotic resident contains only delusion or unreality? How does she know that her unconscious is not similarly deluding her by posing as God? The point is that Joan can make no such distinction with confidence. Indeed, she realizes ironically that people in her profession would see her views as delusional. Thus she drives this conceptual wedge between her "sane" and residents' "insane" unusual experiences in order to stave off this threat of closet insanity.

This threat also underlies staff's typical reluctance to dig into the content of their unusual experiences unless asked to do so through devices like my interviews. Staff would prefer to keep such experiences safely locked up and undisturbed in the closet—thus their fearful ambivalence when probed. Although staff use psychiatric terms to refer to their own experiences—self-label in accord with reverse role modeling—they typically only do so obliquely (and vicariously), while keeping their main focus on the residents. But this strategy ironically backfires because it amplifies reverse role modeling and, ultimately, heightens fear of closet insanity on this basis.

And so staff continually prune both their own and the residents' unusual experiences of all potentially threatening foliage until only the stark and barren trunk of biology remains to distinguish "us" from "them." Kris' account is particularly telling in this regard. This man is deeply imbued with the elegant and profound beauty of the Buddhist tradition. But in his account here this usually perceptive and sensitive soul is transformed into a hard-nosed psychobiologist.

What is the basis of this change? EPIC staff are recruited from and reflect a politically and religiously liberal area of California. Virtually all staff are humanistically oriented and motivated people whose empathy and altruism are the antithesis of the punitive *Cuckoo's Nest* mind-set. Nonetheless, the examples of Kris, Joan, and the others highlight the power of psychiatric ideology to insinuate itself into the core of staff's thinking as at once the ironic source of and solution to insanity. Further, despite whatever beliefs or values psychiatric workers hold, religious or otherwise, the structural role requirements of their job (which will be discussed in Chapters 4 and 5) require that they bow deeply toward psychiatry's central icon and legitimating ideology: the medical disease model (see Chapter 1).[3]

This model firmly plants the allegedly inferior coping and incompetence of labeled psychotics in the "objective" soil of inferior biology, and, as corrollary, plants staff's allegedly superior coping and competence in the "objective" soil of superior biology. (Incidentally, all forms of racism also invoke biology to justify moral superiority.) An Orwellian image comes to mind: "All animals are equal, but some animals (staff) are more equal than others [labeled psychotics] (Orwell 1954:148).

Thus staff feel continually compelled to patrol and shore up the "border." They take pains to portray themselves as more effective, more competent, more valid, more rational—in sum, more normal than the residents, with biology forming the ultimate line of defense. In Chapters 4 and 5 we will explore how this ideology is enacted in practice, but first let us examine the instructive account of the "chief" of the "border patrol," EPIC psychiatrist Dr. Robert Williams.

Chief of Police

An extensive excerpt from my interview with Dr. Williams follows. Although only two psychiatrists were interviewed (I also interviewed Dr. Ogden, who was introduced in Chapter 2), the similarities in their accounts regarding the construction of psychiatric ideology are telling in terms of our analysis of staff as a whole.

BL: By your standards and values, or by your own understanding of your own day-to-day consciousness, have you ever had what you would call an unusual experience or altered state of mind? By that I mean some state of consciousness, behavior, or feelings which departed from your everyday perception in some extreme way for you?

Dr. W: Extreme way? Is the word "extreme"?

BL: Yeah, I think that's important, because I'm asking if there's a "break" from your ordinary frame of reference in some way that's very different for you.

Dr. W: I would say no—not if you use the word "extreme."

BL: If I don't use the word "extreme"?

Dr. W: Yeah, I would say "mild." Yes.

BL: Could you elaborate what a mild departure would be for you?

Dr. W: Sure. If I've had one or two drinks, I get light-headed. If I smoke marijuana, I feel a little funny—little sorts of mild states. There's also a mild state kind of between waking and sleeping in which you kind of experience a free-floating pattern of associations different than one experiences while totally in the waking state.

BL: That free-floating pattern of associations, do you remember any of the visual imagery or anything concretely from those states?

Dr. W: I don't remember anything specifically.

BL: Is there anything about the light-headedness while drinking, or feeling funny that you mentioned happens with marijuana, that you could be more specific about—memory traces, feelings at the time, etc.?

Dr. W: People respond differently. People get detached, a good feeling, a sleepy feeling, sometimes dull feelings, transient access to associations one normally doesn't have access to.

BL: Could you describe more specifically anything you remember about these feelings for you—or this "transient access to associations one normally doesn't have access to"? What's that like for you?

Dr. W: I can't recall any specifics.

BL: In relation to marijuana, one thing that's come up so far in people's answers is often a heightened sense of threat. Do you feel that or any kind of fear state?

Dr. W: No.

BL: I'd like to ask you what these moderately altered states mean to you.

Dr. W: Mildly altered states.

BL: I'm sorry, mildly altered states. What's your sense of what they are or mean to you? The "alteration": What's the source of it, and what sense do you make of it when you're in it?

Dr. W: Oh, I think that they're the product of the effect of the drugs on the central nervous system.

Psychiatrists are the arbiters of what constitutes insanity or sanity in our culture. As chief gatekeepers charged with keeping these realms distinctly separate, they might aptly be called "reality police."[4] As such, Dr. Williams does not want to reveal anything about himself that might suggest, not least to himself, that he is anything but in constant touch with "reality"—is normal by his own psychiatric definition. Thus Dr. W, as chief psychiatric expert, rejects my construction of his unusual experiences as extreme. He insists that I define his unusual experiences as mild instead of extreme. His emphasis on this distinction suggests that, just like subordinate staff, he fears our talk is a diagnostic interview in reverse. Thus he closes the door against the potential negative labeling he associates with "extreme."

As master of this territory, he deflects my probes as deftly as he ordinarily detects symptoms: My question probes Dr. W's prior disclosure that drinking and marijuana induced "mild states" in him. He at once corrects my mistaken reference to his self-defined "mildly altered states" as "moderately altered." And although he indicates that a "free-floating pattern of associations" is part of these experiences, he provides no specifics. Dr. W's vigilant insistence that no definitions of his unusual experiences beyond mild are acceptable and his unwillingness to specify any details of these states underscore that he implicitly constructs our talk as a reverse diagnostic interview.

Further, Dr. W's definition of the interview situation drastically departs from mine. In all the interviews I explain that I am using "extreme" or "unusual" as terms that are entirely *relative* to that particular person's view of his/her ordinary experience as baseline. I take pains to make clear that I see these terms as utterly self-referential. I in no way intend these terms as ordinal variables for ranking an individual's experiences on some objective scale. Nor are they intended as an evaluational measure of "pathology."

But within his projected model of the reverse diagnostic interview, Dr. W implicitly places himself in the role of labeled psychotic. As such he guards against his fearful expectation that I shall diagnose his "symptoms" in accord with some category of psychiatric pathology—as indicated by his response to my use of the term "extreme." Thus seated in the wrong chair, so to speak, Dr. W joins subordinate staff in engaging in reverse role modeling:

BL: Is there anything about the light-headedness while drinking, or feeling
         funny that you mentioned happens with marijuana, that you could be
         more specific about—memory traces, feelings at the time, etc.?
Dr. W: People respond differently. People get detached, a good feeling, a
         sleepy feeling, sometimes dull feelings, transient access to associations
         one normally doesn't have access to.

Dr. W. again ignores the self-referential intent of my probes. Instead, he takes flight into an objectivistically conceived framework of abstract categories of "people," excluding himself and *his* feelings. Dr. W retreats to this detached and aloof vantage point as a defense against my self-referential questions in his projected context of reverse role modeling (which, as we have seen, exacerbates the threat of closet insanity).

Within Dr. W's psychiatric context of meaning, which in good positivist fashion he sees as objective, the term "extreme" no doubt connotes psychosis. Indeed, his model requires that he conflate ordinary terms for psychic states like "extreme," "mild," and "moderate" within a binary normal/abnormal grid. If "extreme" equals "psychotic" in this scheme, perhaps "moderate" equals "neurotic." In any case, Dr. W's insistence on "mild" as the only acceptable alternative among these terms suggests that he sees it as the only opinion on the normal side of the fence.

If Dr. W were to admit to extreme or moderate departures from his everyday experience, this admission would indicate to him that he is neurotic or psychotic—in a word, abnormal. Since his binary model allows for no other opinion, he must deny the use of "extreme" and "moderate" for his experiences. It is his way to ensure the presentation of a normal public persona in his own eyes—and thus ward off any suggestion of hidden or closet insanity. Further, as added self-protection he reduces even his "mild" experiences to a biochemistry bereft of specific detail and his responsible agency:

BL: The 'alteration': What's the source of it, and what sense do you make of it when you're in it?

Dr. W: Oh, I think that they're the product of the effect of the drugs on the central nervous system.

Dr. W ends where his psychiatric ideology begins—in biology. He thus precipitates the living plenitude into a fossilized chemistry as sole explanation. But in its unwillingness to allow for the potential viability and value of alternative realities, psychiatry becomes an ersatz totalitarian religion employed as a rigid and narrow defense against the threat of the unknown. As a "high priest" of psychiatry, Dr. W refuses to interrupt the exclusive sway of its dogma long enough to look anew at his own and labeled-psychotic residents' intimate states of being. Dr. W's account is devoid of critical self-awareness. Simply, he has become the victim of his psychiatric idol.

One sees Dr. W, the consummate psychiatrist, experiencing no extremes. One sees no room in him for visible fear, certainly none for overt disorientation, and none even for sharp questions of his taken-for-granted psychiatric world. He cannot cast into doubt his public persona, cemented as it is, statue like, within psychiatric ideology. His is a seamless world without ruptures. Perhaps the matter is as anthropologist Evans-Pritchard said of the Azande: "He cannot think his thought is wrong."[5] Maybe Dr. W cannot think his thought is wrong without imminent threat to his very existence. Thus he protests too much the "mildness" of his departures from the ordinary: In this virtuoso performance, the consummate psychiatrist becomes the consummate psychiatric border patrolman—while the smell of fear remains.

Notes

1. The educational achievement breakdown among staff is: masters degree or higher=7; bachelor's degree=14; high school only=2; 2 years of college without degree's=5. Thus staff are overwhelmingly college educated. The basic (modal)

requirement for EPIC employment—unless offset by extensive experience in the field—is a bachelor's degree or better, typically in psychology (10) or the social sciences and humanities.

In marked contrast, only two labeled psychotics have college degrees, 17 attended college, with 11 reporting two years or more. Eleven did not even make it through high school.

2.   I attempted to convey not that I was "neutral" in the objectivistic sense of the Olympian observer, the positivist fallacy, but rather in the sense of taking a dispassionate and nonpartisan role during ongoing definitional disputes in the setting. My retrospective analysis, however, takes a partisan stance regarding the central power relation in psychiatric work.

3.   However, there is precious little scientific evidence to support this faith. See especially Sarbin and Mancuso (1980) and Abrams and Taylor (1983), who contend that the application of the disease model to schizophrenia is woefully unscientific according to psychiatry's own premises.

4.   This image is from the title of Anthony Brandt's book, *Reality Police: The Experience of Insanity in America* (1975).

5.   Edward E. Evans-Pritchard, commenting on witchcraft, writes (Evans-Pritchard 1937:194): "In this web of belief every strand depends on every other strand, and Azande cannot get out of its meshes because it is the only world he knows. The web is not an external structure in which he is enclosed. It is the texture of his thought and he cannot think his thought is wrong."

Chapter 4

BORDER LINES

We have seen that staff's psychological vulnerability as role models of sanity is heightened by the daily presense of the labeled-psychotic residents. Staff come to see, fearfully, that their own private problematic experiences could be viewed or termed as identical to those publicly displayed by the residents. In short, closet insanity (the hidden fear that staff might be labeled in the same way as residents) is amplified by reverse role modeling—or the private identification of staff with residents. The upshot of this situation is that staff use their psychiatric ideology to reinforce the threatened psychological border between themselves and residents.

Here this theme will be further elaborated through an analysis directly comparing, on the one hand, both groups' unusual experiences and, on the other, their often conflicting constructions of the location and character of the border. This analysis will emphasize an examination of staff's *interpersonal* strategies for warding off the threat of closet insanity, and will also augment the account of their *ideological* strategies as discussed in the previous chapter. We will also see how these interpersonal strategies form the foundation of the workaday world in the psychiatric enterprise.

Painted Black

Let us begin with a series of unusual experiences. The identity (staff or labeled psychotic) of each excerpt will be temporarily concealed:

Number 1: I heard voices and felt a strange paranoia all the time. I was lethargic. I was very depressed, slightly suicidal, miserable. The voices were flat, the words unintelligible. I heard my name called. A few of the words they said I heard in my head repeatedly. They were unintelligible, but somehow weirdly familiar and known to me. But I couldn't repeat them to people. I felt real dead and blank. I had a flat affect when I talked.

Number 2:   I saw mountains of vomit and people's dismembered bodies, excretions, and slime—mountains of it. And vile animals. I felt like throwing up. I felt I was a black spot on the face of the earth: Piles of dirt in the universe on snow-covered land. My breath would get short, and if I wanted to I could die. You can will yourself to death. I felt a knife would go through me. Sometimes I'm real paranoid. I feel people plotting. Nobody cares and everybody hates me. I'm a martyr of the universe to be singled out and tortured in some freak way. I felt I was the girl with no eyes. I felt everybody thought that about me.

Number 3:   My depression feels like a blanket, not only mental but physical. If I lay on my bed, I feel like I am sinking through the bed. I have to hide and get suicidal. I start drinking, and when I'm depressed I get real high. Sometimes I get so high or depressed the only relief is to drink or carve on my wrist. This is sick, honest! When I get depressed and get in a blanket, I get somewhere else. I feel out of control. I am out of myself so much, it's like reviewing a movie of what I did later.

Number 4:   When I'm depressive, I have feelings of hopelessness, despair, no way out—physical and emotional sickness. I get nervous stomach, nausea, sleeplessness. I isolate myself, become nonverbal, even suicidal.

Number 5:   I was at the point of being so depressed that I had a distorted view of everything—not out of touch, but very distorted. Everything in life, internal and external, seemed completely and absolutely negative, depressing, and hopeless. These painful feelings of depression seemed unchangeable.

Number 6:   I had much depression—suicide attempts which lasted over most of my teenage years. My depression was so pervasive it affected my complete outlook. It led to breakdown of my perceptual abilities: Not acute psychosis, but my paranoia had some schizy qualities. [I ask him to elaborate what he means by the latter.] No hallucinations or delusions—though I thought people were talking about me. I stayed in a room for three weeks out of fear of others. Not physical, but emotional fear.

Emotional pain is a dominant theme in all the accounts. But alongside this thematic unity, there is one striking contrast: Numbers 1, 5, and 6 (Lela, Nadine, and Nigel) speak of their dark times in the past tense, whereas numbers 3 and 4 (Maude and Nanette) express their pain in the present tense. (Let us skip number 2 momentarily.) In fact, this contrast enables us to choose the correct identity of each excerpt: The former are staff, the latter residents.

Beyond this difference, there is little that distinguishes these accounts. Psychiatric terms like "paranoid," "depression," "depressive," "schizy," and (the more generic) "sick" pepper both groups' references to their experiences. Thus, as reverse role modeling would predict, staff join residents in "psychiatrizing" their experiences.

Why do staff speak of these experiences in the past tense, while residents locate them in the present? We have already seen that staff are societal gatekeepers charged with keeping the realms of sanity and insanity strictly separate ideologically and practically. This status requires that staff be public arbiters and role models of social and psychological health and competence. But reverse role modeling leads staff to identify their problematic private experiences with the similar public experiences of the labeled-psychotic residents. Since staff must maintain their status as healthy role models, they must keep these experiences mostly hidden. In this case, after having revealed and labeled these dark experiences, staff close the closet door and turn the light on. In other words, they tell us, society, that these labeled events are a thing of the past—painful learning experiences that have been outgrown and are now defunct.

Staff ward off the deepening threat that closet insanity and reverse role modeling pose to their public status as psychiatric workers. The labeled-psychotic residents, however, by definition the current occupants of certified insane status, are under no such constraints to distance themselves from their psychological pain. In fact, it is the essential condition of their status. And while the mental hospital and EPIC clientele at first resist psychiatric labels, they most often come to embrace and identify with this negative status—even using it (and suicidal threats) to gain entry into what has become for them a home away from home (see Chapter 2).

Let us now return to excerpt number 2. Psychiatric ideology would certainly frame these darkly grotesque experiences as hallucinatory and delusional, as—in a word—psychotic. But Tammy is neither a labeled psychotic nor a staff person. Rather, she is a successful science fiction writer with no history of affiliation with the psychiatric enterprise.

Since Tammy is apparently well-adapted to the demands of legitimate society, her psychic reality, though seemingly strange and painful, is unlikely to be subject to psychiatric intervention. Thus psychiatric criteria are unlikely to be applied to her experiences. Although Tammy is my only nonpsychiatric interviewee, my hunch is that bizarre imagery can at one time or other inhabit the mental ecology of almost anyone. But without the psychiatric context of meaning, off-beat experiences usually do not get crystallized as evidence of psychosis.

Nevertheless, Tammy self-labels much like staff, using the term "paranoid" for her experiences (although unlike staff she is unfamiliar with psychiatric settings, and therefore shows no fear of the dangers of labeling). If psychiatric labels are not readily applied to people outside the psychiatric context, then why does Tammy self-label? This phenomenon may suggest that the psychiatric industry has successfully indoctrinated people through the mass media and culture industry to use psychiatric terms to refer to their emotional difficulties. In any case, future research on the extent to which psychiatric ideology has penetrated everyday references to personal problems might be of consequence. (Are labeled psychotics becoming reverse role models for everybody?)

Not of This World

Let us explore another series of unusual experiences. Again, the staff or labeled-psychotic identity of each excerpt is temporarily concealed:

Number 1: I was in a room alone meditating, and opened my eyes to the presence of spiritual people with me. They weren't clear like you there. I opened my eyes to circles of people in the room talking about me, but I couldn't hear them. It was psychic stuff. I know I wasn't shielded enough. I was frightened because I was unprepared and not guarded enough. . . . It's like dealing with spirits of some altered state a being is in. . . . I see myself as a Dianic witch and pagan—a woman-centered, woman-goddess identity. I do rituals and ceremonies like that. I believe in reincarnation and altered states of psychic ability; out of body experiences. I can more or less do that at will. I can't control it after I've left my body, but I have the ability to put myself in a trance enabling it to happen. I've had memories of previous lives. I know I lived in the time when the persecution of witches occurred, and that I died twice. I am a powerful, gentle witch who practices witchcraft and goddess worship and nature worship.

Number 2: My body would move, walk around, sit with everyone, have a conversation. But my heart, soul, and mind would leave my body and look down at myself and people around. [At this point she gets up and walks across the room, then looks back at the empty chair as if at a palpable presence.] I do this and look back at myself in the chair—it happens outside my body. One part of me gets up and leaves, then leans back and takes a look at everything I'm saying and doing. [Her face assumes a faraway look as she stares into the corner of the room and says, "I think I can do it now."] I just did it: A transparent invisible me went over there, and looked in the window and in the corner, getting different views instead of one.

Number 3:　My friend and I were rafting in white water in the Feather River in winter and went over twelve-foot falls into the water. I yelled out—but without a voice—"We're dead," and he yelled back—without a voice— "I know." It's the same as people describing your whole life flashing before you: I was a kid on a bike, back in my marriage. I could live in all planes in time at once. I was in the seat of power. . . . I could trace the floating of my body twenty miles downstream, and I could feel my friend's body downstream, too. In the seat of power, with both of us dead, we could think together even though we were both dead. In death we simultaneously decided to go back to school and live life over again. Just then I got back in my body and pulled myself up onto the raft with a rope. My friend did that too. We were heading for other falls, and I grabbed a willow branch. We reached shore and crawled to the car. I felt the intense pain of thawing out by the car heater. We died in a hundred other worlds. We saw news articles about our deaths. . . . We went to a restaurant, and the walls of the place were full of news clippings about people who died in the water during winter. The local people there said, "You couldn't survive falling into the water in winter."

But there are multiple universes. There are lots of earths like this where I definitely died and went on as dead, but was launched into another material world—here—where time and space is zero. It doesn't exist. I'm back in this world where we're talking. You just pick and choose among infinite worlds. It's a religious belief. I think people who are diagnosed schizophrenic think they are dead and have given up bodily life. If they were there, in an alternative universe, they wouldn't be able to talk right. It would be a "word salad" because they would be talking to many different people at once. Word salad is the simultaneity of different worlds.

Number 4:　When I play my music and paint, it isn't me, but channeling from some higher place. I am a free spirit who gets inner messages from my third eye opening up. I am one of 144,000 chosen people on the planet trying to get to the New Age of Wisdom. I am one of the prophets receiving messages from on high, from God. I've been around the universe four times to try to bring about a healing, but it can't be done by myself alone. Everyone who is chosen has a spiritual awakening. Then we find out what our work is on this planet. We are the nomads of the world. We all have our assignments. We know where to go and what to do because we are guided people.

I have given myself to the work of God that needs to be done on this planet. This planet is rocking and out of balance, and so are most of its people. If these things stay out of balance, I can't tell you what will happen, except we the chosen will be the only ones left. Those in power cannot and do not want to help the helpless. I am identified with all people, and all people can reach potentials much greater than they think. You never want anyone to have power

Number 5:   I receive thoughts which I feel are a gift from outside me, rather
than from my own consciousness. There's a sensation of energy
moving through my body, a physical sensation, and extending out
of my body—particularly my hands. I receive guidance on personal questions from a higher source: Simply, open surrender to
whatever happens, to God. I ask God what it's like to get "yes,"
and ask what happens. Then I ask what it's like to get "no." I can
ask questions of God and get answers through my body with
prearranged signals as to what "yes" and "no" is. But the goal is
the unconscious source of information—God. There's a sense of
union with higher powers. These bodily states are sources of
teaching or information from the unconscious, which is God, and
sometimes it erupts into consciousness. I do a lot of meditation,
trying to be open to the will of God. These experiences function as
goals to be worked toward, a sense of what is possible.

Numbers 1 and 5 (Karla and Joan) are staff; numbers 2, 3, and 4
(Simone, Richard, and Kate) are labeled psychotics. How accurate is your
diagnostic judgment this time? Both residents and staff tell stories of
previous lives, fantastic identities, out-of-body experiences, otherworldly presences, alternative universes—in short, various altered states
of mind and existence. Interestingly, staff do not banish these accounts to
the past, as they did their tales of dark times, but join residents in framing
them in the present. In fact, besides the more dramatic quality of
residents' imagery, there is little that distinguishes the contents of these
accounts.

But one contrast is telling. In order not to give away the identity of the
staff excerpts, I deleted background details that typically appear alongside staff's other-worldly claims. For example, Karla intersperses these
comments in her story:

I'm real cautious about revealing unusual states, because I have no evidence
to justify them to peers. . . . I know it's confidential, but I'm afraid. . . . It's
separate from my mental health work. . . . There's a stigma.

And Joan adds this disclaimer to her account:

Most psychiatrists, even most of my profession [Joan has a Ph.D. in
psychology] still see this stuff as crazy—they're so unspiritual—so I keep it
under wraps a lot. [She laughs.] This *is* confidential!

Thus the major substantive differences between the accounts of the two groups is the fact that staff typically pepper their stores with asides expressing anxiety or rationalizations, while residents do not. Staff tales are told with a self-reflexive caution missing from the accounts of residents. What is the basis of this contrast? For one thing, as we saw in Chapter 2, the labeled-psychotic role includes the expectation that one's mind appears to be out of control, and accordingly, the ongoing willingness to elaborate "symptoms." And, to add to the earlier point regarding their dark experiences, since labeled psychotics are already certified as insane, they have nothing to lose through public disclosure of fantastic experiences that, indeed, form the second major source of their social status.

Further, although staff self-label as part of identification with residents, that is, engage in reverse role modeling, at the same time the fearful asides and disclaimers are meant to buffer the intensified threat of closet insanity accruing from this process. Staff act preemptively to head off challenges to their status as arbiters of social and psychological competence that they fear could result from such fantastic reports. But this strategy itself emerges from staff's projection of the diagnostic interview onto other social settings and, therefore, ironically, also reflects reverse role modeling.

The question remains as to why staff report their uncorroborated experiences in the present, albeit with trepidation, while referring their dark experiences to the past. Part of the answer may lie outside the psychiatric context per se, and may reflect a more general cultural reality. My belief is that revelation of seemingly out-of-control or unresolved emotional difficulties is more stigmatized in this culture than is the disclosure of altered states of mind and existence. While the former may indicate to many people a weakness of character in coping with life's knocks, the latter can convey a sense of romantic adventure—the notion of conquest of "inner space" and the like.

Applying this insight to the analysis so far, it was suggested in Chapter 2 that the anarchically freewheeling and direct communication of labeled psychotics is one attraction of psychiatric work. It could be that this romantic dimension of "mad talk" is bound up with reverse role modeling in the sense that staff not only unconsciously but actively and consciously emulate it. In the context of their workaday world, a discussion of the more culturally accepted altered states of mind becomes paradoxically less stigmatizing for staff.

A central issue in the above excerpts involves the relative influence of content vs. context regarding the labeling of uncorroborated claims. For example, both (R) Kate and (S) Joan claim to communicate directly with God. Kate says that her art and spiritual insight are not she, but "channeling from some higher place," i.e., "from God," and similarly,

Joan contends that the deity directly provides guidance on "personal questions" by sending "prearranged signals" through her body.

While the contents of both claims are similarly fantastic, their respective social character and purpose are decidedly different. Kate's account emphasizes her desire to heal the planet and save our species from planetary catastrophe—to usher in the "New Age of Wisdom." Kate fuses religious and political images in a prophetic ethical critique of modern civilization, and calls for social and otherworldly transformation on this basis. Unlike Kate, however, Joan claims no special mission in God's service to heal the world. There is no explicit social vision for the reform or enrichment of the human condition. On the contrary, Joan's "sense of union with higher powers" seemingly focuses divine intervention only on her own personal issues.

The substance of Joan's account reveals an individualistic and even solipsistic preoccupation with self. But Kate's altruistic concern and commitment to the planet, while admittedly often delivered in an idiosyncratic idiom, has helped to earn her a designation of psychotic. The point is that the substance of claims—whether fantastic, selfish, or altruistic—is not decisive to the attribution of sanity or insanity. As with the nonpsychiatric case of Tammy, the fate of closely linked experiences of the unusual has much less to do with the nature of their content than with the social context in which they are claimed.

Let us look at another example from outside a psychiatric context of meaning. Consider the noted astronomer Carl Sagan. Certainly he is in no sense considered mad; he is, in fact, a major cultural celebrity. Yet his view of planetary reality is essentially Kate's, without the overt religiosity. His argument, in effect, is precisely that our planet is, as Kate puts it, "rocking and out of balance"—gravely threatened by current productive and environmental practices. And his implicit position is like Kate's in that he sees the "love of power" as underlying much of our planetary madness and plight (Sagan 1985).

While the powers that be do not call Sagan's views insane, they do call them "unrealistic." Carl Sagan avoids the fate of having his ideas discredited as delusions because he has a positive master status as a notable citizen, and delivers his views in public forums entirely outside the psychiatric framework. Nonetheless, Sagan's ideas are to date as ineffectual as Kate's. It matters not that the projection of planetary catastrophe in both accounts may show a deadly accurate grasp of the likely result of the current course of our civilization. At present this position lacks societal agreement and a power base from which to alter our official political policies.

Thus staff (and people at large) often hold views and harbor experiences every bit as fantastic or troublesome as those of labeled psychotics.

Staff know that, given a psychiatric frame of reference, the same labels applied to the residents' experiences could apply to their own. This observation suggests that the "truth" or "falsehood," "sanity" or "insanity" of personal claims and political policies is entirely bound to specific social contexts of meaning. And the different responses to key societal issues likewise depend entirely on the relative power of definition and action of the various groups that contend over them. Thus we find that no ontologically objective basis either for personal or societal sanity exists. The definition of what is sane and insane is thoroughly political—a matter of the definitions of the powerful and the power of definitions.

Psychiatric staff know well the centrality of power in matters of definition. That is why, insofar as staff project a psychiatric context onto social settings outside the workplace (the largely unconscious result of reverse role modeling), they will at the same time erect ideological barriers derived from positivist psychiatry as "objective standards" serving to separate and protect themselves from the residents. Interestingly, these ideological barriers are employed even by those staff who have expressed a distaste for and disbelief in psychiatry. These self-protective walls prove to be an illusion, however (recall Karla's comment, "I'm real cautious about revealing unusual states, because I have no evidence to justify them to peers . . . "), as demonstrated in the previous excerpts when I temporarily deleted the identities of (removed the ideological border between) staff and resident claimants.

And since the border can become a most indistinct place without the psychiatric ideology *outside* the psychiatric workplace, in this case EPIC, we find the application of this ideology particularly important to staff *inside* the workplace. The salient "objective" contrast between staff and residents is that, while staff beliefs remain mostly "closeted" in private contexts, the similar beliefs of residents are parade-marched around the psychiatric setting under the master banner "psychotic." We turn now to explore these processes.

The Joke's on Them

The following excerpts are from staff discussions of the residents while apart from them in the work setting, and include psychological consults and staff meetings.

On Kate

> Craig: She [Kate] wants me to believe in her, and to convert to understand that what she's telling me is what's so.

Dr. W:	She may have to hear that it's not always appropriate to hear that all the time. Some people just don't want to hear it. For example, me. [Laughter.]
Lela:	Does she try to get people to accept it, or does she just ventilate it?
Cathy:	[Sings,] "This is the dawning of the age of Aquarius" [Laughter.]
Dr. W:	Actually, I'm not very interested in it.
Clara:	You're not a New Age person? [Wild laughter.]
Cathy:	[Mock serious tone,] So who is responsible for mowing the lawn and killing all the angels in the grass? [Laughter.]
Craig:	Somebody is! [Laughter.]
Cathy:	There are schizophrenics, and there are schizophrenics. I hate every one of them that's here.

Craig observes that Kate is trying to convert him to her beliefs. (We recall Kate as the woman who believes she is on a mission from God to heal the planet.) We might consider that her proselytizing mimics the psychiatric industry's like attempt to convert everybody under its sway to psychiatric ideology: At all points in the psychiatric apparatus—from police car to hospital suite—residents are indoctrinated with the ideology that they are mentally ill and in need of psychiatric expertise to treat it. So viewed, Craig's statement about Kate can be turned on its head to read: Psychiatry "wants . . . to convert [everybody] to understand that what [it's] telling [them] is what's so." In this regard, no doubt many residents would also apply Dr. W's sentiments about Kate's beliefs to his own ideology, namely, that they "don't want to hear it."

Cathy keys to fellow staff's opening observations by satirizing Kate's religiosity: Her singing joke about the "dawning of the age of Aquarius" aims to discredit Kate's position. Dr. W follows Cathy's lead with deadpanned disinterest in Kate's views, whereupon Clara joins the degradation ceremony with her droll rhetorical question as to whether Dr. W is a "New Age person." Clara's ironic pose here reflects her knowledge that Dr. W is not only a nonbeliever, but in fact diagnosed Kate as psychotic precisely on the basis of her religious claims.

Cathy goes on to mock Kate's concern with the fate of the "angels in the grass." Here we notice the fundamental clash between Kate's religious faith in "things unseen" and the staff's professed (at work, anyway) positivist faith in the "facts" underpinning psychiatry. But in this duel of dogmas, psychiatry has the last laugh: Cathy's parting comment about hating schizophrenics, delivered with self-consciously exaggerated pique, rounds out staff's tragicomic negation of Kate's reality.

On Vern

Cathy:	Vern still has periods where he'll stand out in the backyard on one foot, like a crane. He's very slow, staring off into the Netherlands.

[Cathy stares into space with a mockingly blank expression as staff laugh.]

Ken: It's like yogic exercises.

Clara: Like slow-motion t'ai chi [Chinese exercises], if you could imagine that.

Craig: Jonathan Livingston Schizophrenic![1] [Wild laughter.]

Nadine: He prefers to watch TV when it's snowy rather than clear. I don't know what it means. [She rolls her eyes as staff chuckle.]

Cathy: Well, if he ever turns around and goes [she feigns a high-pitched voice] "they're here"—you'd better watch it. [Wild laughter; this is a reference to a scene in the film *Poltergeist*.]

Clara: And we can't find him! I'm not staying around the house, OK?

Cathy: Vern has got to get clearer so we can talk to him. He's never been like this. He was mute and catatonic here before, but emerged out of it. This is a real tough cookie. Maybe we can take him to somebody who'll pretend to be a Zen master. Maybe Kate [a resident who is a self-proclaimed prophet] would do it! [Laughter.]

Melissa: [In a serious tone,] Maybe we could put him with somebody and keep him with that person and nobody else.

Cathy: Along with a big bottle of Navane! [Antipsychotic drug; laughter.]

Cathy caricatures Vern's physical stance in meditation as cranelike, and pejoratively mimics his state of mind as blank while so involved. (We recall Vern's spiritually based opposition to psychiatric drugs.) Ken and Clara then satirize Vern's pose as forms of exotic (and implicitly symptomatic) exercise, with Craig delivering the labeling punchline "Jonathan Livingston Schizophrenic" to uproarious staff laughter. Nadine and Cathy continue the levity by playing off a scene from *Poltergeist*, a popular horror film in which a modern household is invaded by otherworldly forces via the television, with Vern the ghostly main character in their version.

Then the talk turns suddenly serious as Cathy labels Vern's state of mind "mute and catatonic"—a distinctive indicator of the diagnosis of schizophrenia. In this connection, maybe the taciturn Vern is avoiding talk—the stuff of symptoms—in order to prevent his deeper entanglement in the psychiatric net as "Jonathan Livingston Schizophrenic."

After showing marked frustration with Vern's lack of progress within the psychiatric enterprise, Cathy jokes about linking him up with the self-proclaimed prophet Kate as "Zen master." Cathy's comedic discrediting of Vern's and Kate's spiritual preoccupations thus hits two labeled psychotic birds with one psychiatric stone. But Cathy's final joke shows where a perplexed psychiatry, a most un–Zen-like discipline, turns to as both first and last resort to secure its ideological supremacy: "a big bottle of Navane" (the drug) as she puts it.

On Kay

> *Craig:*   I said to Kay, "Why did Dr. W. increase your meds?" Then she
>   answered, "Well, I had a glass of wine this weekend, and maybe he did
>   it because of that." [Craig's voice then deepens and gets loud.] So she
>   hasn't any idea, or insight.
>   Clara, Cathy, Larry, and Ken: [Chant as chorus,] Nooo. [Laughter.]
> *Cathy:*   [Imitates a mechanical, robotlike voice,] Null and void. [Laughter.]
> *Craig:*   [He picks up a tennis racket; then, while looking coolly at it, says,] She
>   probably can't even see to the bottom of my grip.

Acting as straight man, Craig soberly discredits Kay's explanation that
a "glass of wine" is responsible for her increased regimen of drugs as lack
of "insight" into her condition ("insight" presumably meaning Kay's
acknowledgment that she requires the larger dosage for her worsening
mental illness). Suitably cued, the other staff chant the punch line "Nooo"
as an ironic Greek chorus echoing Craig's devaluation of Kay's definition
of her situation. Amid staff laughter, Cathy likens Kay to a vacuous
automaton without independent intelligence: "Null and void." Finally,
Craig coolly rounds out this sketch with his image of Kay's alleged
inability to perceive his "grip" (on sanity) on the tennis racket.

Hardly the blind robot that Craig and Cathy have constructed, Kay
does not seriously believe that her recent glass of wine is the real reason
for the change in her drug regimen. Rather, her comment more plausibly
indicates an insightful satire of the overuse of psychiatric drugs for
behavioral control, and the blind and arbitrary raising and lowering of
dosage on this basis. Further, it suggests that the psychiatric taboo
against labeled psychotics' use of recreational drugs is hypocritical
(especially in light of the fact that residents suffer so many untoward
effects from the prescribed and forced psychiatric variety). In sum, Kay is
very much aware of Craig and company's "grip," and acts to loosen it by
having—as many of us do, including Dr. W—an occasional glass of wine.

On Lyndon

> *Craig:*   Lyndon actually volunteered something in group.
> *Cathy:*   [With mock incredulousness,] Honest to God:
> *Craig:*   Yep. He said he couldn't do the dishes because he had "psychoemo-
>   tional experiences." I don't know what that means, but he used those
>   words. I asked Lyndon whether there was any way he could commu-
>   nicate to his peers how these psychoemotional experiences keep him
>   from doing the dishes. [Staff begin to chuckle.] And he said, "I don't
>   know if I can do that." I said that if he could communicate about it, it

might help because people were irritated that he didn't do the dishes. I asked him if it was OK if people in the group could ask him if he had psychoemotional experiences.

Lela: [Seriously,] Could he define it?

Craig: Yes, he could. I asked him if he was hallucinating or hearing voices, but he wouldn't call it that, or talk about anything he was preoccupied with. He didn't want to call it anything else except psychoemotional experiences. [Staff laughter increases.] But he could define it: He said that it's when he's spaced out and can't focus in on anything—when he can't focus in on concrete things. It's when he can't do the task at hand, because he's so removed from that. He says, 'I keep being pulled away,' but wouldn't say why.

Ken: I have to go have a "psychoemotional experience"—I have to go "pee." [He deadpans to wild laughter.]

Craig again acts as straight man. He reports, with an air reserved for momentous occasions, that Lyndon "actually" took autonomous action. So cued, Cathy deepens Craig's satirical gambit with mock disbelief at his "startling" revelation. After Lela asks seriously whether Lyndon can define "psychoemotional experiences," Craig outlines the ways in which he does so amid growing staff laughter.

Lyndon resists the imposition of psychiatric ideology by rejecting Craig's terms for his experiences, "hallucinating" or "hearing voices," which are consistent with a diagnosis of schizophrenia. Instead, he coins his own psychiatric term and clearly defines its meaning as his inability to focus on anything concrete or do instrumental tasks because he is "pulled away" from them when "so removed" by these experiences. Staff amusement notwithstanding, Lyndon's term better fits the practical impact these experiences have on his everyday life than does the standard psychiatric fare. But in the end the psychiatric power of definition prevails, as indicted by Ken's final satiric parry, "I have to go 'pee,' " which crudely trivializes Lyndon's term. Staff discredit Lyndon's attempt to define his situation to his own satisfaction by rendering it absurd and illusory.

We have thus seen staff often using dark humor to gang up rhetorically on residents. Why do staff, for the most part empathetic individuals who deeply care about others' well-being, engage in this activity? Faced daily with the public emotional pain of labeled residents, staff are threatened by their growing identification with this pain, which intensifies their own (de)pressing private problems and experiences. In sum, reverse role modeling heightens the fear of closet insanity and, in psychological terms, generates cognitive dissonace. And one major sociological escape route from the personal anxiety (cognitive dissonance) created by reverse role modeling is the role distance provided by dark humor. And this "symptomatic" relief can only be had at the expense of the official occupants of the labeled-psychotic status.

Thus staff send up clouds of cynical jokes as a major self-protective smoke screen to hide and buffer their intensifying closet insanity. The central sociological function of the comedic degradation ceremonies built into psychiatric work is to enforce the illusion of radical separation between "sane" and "insane" worlds—and this defensive camouflage often turns darker still. We turn now to explore these processes.

Boy Are They Crazy

The following excerpts, like the previous series, are also from staff discussions of residents while apart from them in the work setting:

On Erin

Cathy: As far as social agreements we make with people, Erin does want to please, get along, but he does weird things. He pets me on the head! [Laughter.] I'm making tuna salad, and he's petting me on the head, saying, "I wish I had long hair like yours." I said, "Erin, you're petting me on the head," and then he says, "I had hair 19 inches long once." I asked whether that was in his old hippie days, and [Cathy screws up her face in mock incomprehension] he looked at me like I had just said something in Hebrew to him, like [mock incredulousness] "old hippie days?" [Staff laughter grows.] I said, "Don't pet me on the head, tell me you like me." [Wild laughter.]

Karla: He says things to me like, "I'd rather be a Maytag," or, "My mom's German shepherd worries about me too much"—things with meaning only to Erin. [Laughter.] There's a kernel of truth there somewhere, but I can't find it.

Larry: There are periods where he's lucid and really together: All of the word salad and weirdness, talk of Hitler, and quantum physics is gone. Then he goes off meds, and spends two years tyring to get back again.

Craig: When was the last time he was clear, 1960? [Laughter.]

Cathy: He helped rebuild his mom's house two years ago, so what does every good chronic do?

Larry: Hey, I don't need my meds anymore!

Cathy: Yup, and he plummeted rapidly, and has never come back since.

Clara: He told (S) Melissa, after coming on to her sexually, that "I wash my hands after I defecate." That's a real sexual kind of line! [Laughter and groans.]

Craig: Erin washes his hands after somebody *else* defecates! [Wild laughter.]

Larry: He just can't do it, he can't function interpersonally. He's just an idiot! [Wild laughter continues.] He made a good contract yesterday [Larry's voice is exasperated]: "Go to volunteer work;" "Participate in groups;" "Do chores." But even if he does everything, I can't see them [the people at the cheap hotel where Erin is likely to be placed after discharge from EPIC] accepting him. He'll look at the manager and say, "My mother breast-fed me." [Wild laughter.]

Erin's head-petting suggests that Erin wantonly breaks most of the rules of face-to-face communication. And, as Goffman (1971:335–390) points out, exactly such disruptive behavior leads to social exclusion in the first place. The assembled staff proceed to catalog Erin's numerous interactional gaffes with a strangely bittersweet mix of frustrated concern and amused chagrin.

I emphasize that my point in highlighting these staff descriptions of residents' behavior is *not* that they are fabricated by staff, or that the behavior described would not be viewed as "strange" in the everyday world. Rather, the central issue is that staff use these descriptions to cope with their own fears about "sanity." This defensive use is further underscored by the fact that staff rarely interpret their observations on residents' behavior as indications of "health."

Staff attribute Erin's return to incompetent behavior after periods of competence to his unwillingness to keep taking the psychiatric drugs that staff see as the source of his competence (indeed, as the only hope for career-labeled psychotics like Erin). However, as outlined in Chapter 2, Erin is trapped in the no-win cultural situation of being stigmatized as "sick" with or without drugs. Thus labeled psychotics often poignantly try to live without the drugs and their side effects.

Staff almost gloat over Erin's and "every good chronic's" failure to function after stopping the drugs as suitable punishment for so transgressing this psychiatric sacrament. And Craig's ironic barb casting doubt on Larry's claim that Erin has ever been "lucid and really together," drugs or no drugs, shows a deep and abiding resentment alongside the usual dark humor.

What makes staff so angry with Erin? Erin's periods of adequate performance suggest at first that staff are successful at their ostensibly rehabilitative craft. These apparent breakthroughs, however, turn out to be short-lived as Erin slides back into his old ways (a typical pattern as we saw in Chapter 2). With their expectations so raised, staff feel betrayed and become self-doubting when, like Erin, residents repeatedly fail. And since staff are genuinely concerned with the well-being of residents and believe that they fully employ their expertise to help them, the impulse to blame them for their failure grows with each new example. (The psychoanalytic concept "countertransference"—in essence the subsequent bullying of those one first tries to help but cannot—is relevant here). The threat to staff identity inherent in this failure to rehabilitate is typically displaced onto the residents who are alleged to sabotage treatment by going off drugs and by making other infractions of psychiatric ideology.

Let us examine Erin's failure by taking a closer look at the nature of his cryptic faux pas: Cathy's comedic gambit on Erin's "head-petting" has a serious underside. This behavior, together with his comment that his mother's German shepherd "worries" about him, conjures a suggestive scenario: Perhaps Erin feels patronized, not unlike a domestic animal, by parental and psychiatric authority. It is plausible that, discredited as a full person in his own right, Erin finds a way to turn the tables on this situation: He pets Cathy's head in order to put her into the patronized and subordinated status usually reserved for him.

Erin's claim that he would "rather be a Maytag" also lends support to this scenario. The reference is to a TV commercial in which a Maytag repairman wears a sad expression because he is lonely. The idea is that Maytag appliances never break down, and therefore the repairman is never called upon to work. Erin's use of this image pointedly speaks to his situation: Unlike Maytag applicances, which (at least according to the ad) are strong and never break down, Erin has repeated breakdowns, which result in his social exclusion. Erin views the Maytag as a kind of mentor. It possesses the strength and invulnerability to manipulation that Erin desires. If Erin emulated this machine, the repairmen (psychiatric workers) would be rendered superfluous. Rather than being the victim of psychiatry and its tools (like drugs), Erin as a Maytag would be valuable to society. Without Erin as labeled psychotic—essentially as broken machine—the psychiatric staff and pharmaceutical companies would, like the Maytag repairman, become dejected over their obsolescence.

The laughing at Erin's antics, like his comments on defecation and handwashing in regard to sexual relations, continues. And staff expect that he will persist in such bizarre behavior once out of their care. But even in the most jumbled "word salad" (Larry's term is often used for labeled psychotics' alleged incomprehensibility) there are clearly discernible vegetables: among these are patronage, subordination, discrediting, rejection, and isolation. The "kernel of truth" Karla looks for in Erin's talk is well-summarized in these words by cultural critic Bertolt Brecht: "He who is still smiling has not heard the bad news."[2]

In light of their own private fears and difficulties in coping with everyday life, staff resentment of the residents' repeated failures to do as staff must do grows apace (see especially Clara's comments in Chapter 3). And insofar as staff come to believe that the reason residents fail is willful avoidance of the task of living, their anger rises precipitously. We find an otherwise democratically minded Larry characterizing Erin as "just an idiot!" As the burden of policing the border and the burdens of everyday life grow, staff's dark humor becomes ever more strained, until all comedic roads end up in the cul de sac of still darker labels.

On Simone

Craig: So Simone's more stable now?
Cathy: She's less psychotic.
Craig: If I talk with her about anything emotional directly, she will talk about Marilyn Monroe or Charles Manson—anything distracting. She totally avoids.
Cathy: With business stuff, government assistance, disability forms, she'll stay with you, but nothing else.
Craig: I hear her talking, even being natural with people, and she talks about Manson's birthday and how she's connected with him, and psychotic stuff like that.
Cathy: This thing about thought broadcasting never goes away—with or without medication. She has this enduring belief in telepathic power. She also paints everybody else black.
Dr. W: Well, she's still paranoid: less so, perhaps, more covered sometimes, but still psychotic.

Craig contends that Simone "avoids" talking about important emotional issues and "distracts" the talk into seemingly irrelevant topics like Marilyn Monroe, Charles Manson, and other "psychotic stuff." Since psychiatry's definition of paranoia is a belief or fear held without basis in reality, staff's account of Simone's preoccupations lack any effort to understand their sources. Instead, much like in the case of Erin's odd utterances, but minus the humor, they are dismissed as symptomatic of psychotic delusion and left at that.

But let us look more closely at Simone's interest in the Manson and Monroe figures: What is the basis of their attraction for her? Having met Simone, I see her as fitting the stereotype of feminine beauty in our culture—as did Monroe. Unfortunately, Simone's social history indicates that she was sexually abused as a child, as was Monroe. Now Simone finds herself called psychotic and housed in a psychiatric setting.

Just reasoning from this information, it is plausible that these characters strike a responsive chord in Simone associated with their respective notorieties as murderously rebellious outsider (Manson) and martyred victim (Monroe). Perhaps Simone sees Manson as exemplary of a violent culture (Archer 1984), which masks its true nature by diverting popular attention to sensational acts of violence. At the same time, this culture ignores the more prosaic but systemic violence that includes the discrediting of people like Simone. (Incidentally, Manson himself has made this implicit sociological argument by calling himself the "product of the middle class.")[3] Further, maybe Simone identifies with Monroe as an exploited woman whose creativity was forced into a procrustean bed (and onto the casting couch) as a fetishized bauble for male consumption.

But the point of my speculative construction here is not to get at the "truth" of Simone's situation, but rather to highlight that, far from "distractions," Simone's preoccupations are key areas for analysis. Such investigations might provide insight into both Simone's pain and our culture's deficiencies and, who knows, might also provide promising avenues for transcending them. However, the raison d'être of psychiatric ideology is precisely not to engage in such inquiries, but rather to obscure these social sources of our individual and collective suffering by reducing them to individual "pathologies."

The assembled staff carry out this task with dispatch: Cathy catalogs Simone's "thought broadcasting" and "belief in telepathic power" as compelling evidence (symptoms) of her psychotic illness, and again pays no attention to the content of these alleged psychic modalities. Indeed, a focus on their content would reveal the essential sameness of Simone's publicly proclaimed uncorroborated claims and staff's privately closeted admissions. Cathy keeps the closet door shut with the light out—then claims that Simone "paints everybody else black." If so, then Simone—much like Erin—only turns the tables on the degradation ceremonies usually aimed at her and her peers. Nevertheless, psychiatry still has the last "black" word: As Dr. W concludes, she is "still psychotic." The border remains secure.

On Vern

Larry: It's too bad the video isn't working.

Cathy: This is the time we need it: When Vern's got bubbles coming out of his fingers, he says, and he's got a halo, and all that weird stuff, and he looks so strange. You know, that, that . . . [Cathy gropes for words, then her talk breaks off into staring as if speechless.]

Craig: Weird! [Strong emphasis.]

Larry: Yeah!

Cathy: He's very strange.

Dr. W: He's got to begin to accept that he's got a major psychotic illness, that he's schizophrenic.

Nadine: I asked Vern what he was thinking about, and he said he was thinking, "People are reading my mind—lots of people." I asked him, "Are they reading your mind, or are you reading your mind?" He said, "I can't talk about it anymore." He says, "I am talking with God," and weak-kneed, asks if he is coming back to the hospital.

Ken: He comes around from that psychotic junk after taking meds.
Cathy: He always says the side effects of meds makes everything worse. It's more than side effects with Vern. He's absolutely adamant about denying. I came right out and said, "When you do this kind of stuff, that's your psychosis." He goes, [Cathy mimics an incredulous look] "Psychosis," and gets upset like he's gonna sue me, and I say, "That's the name you give it, that's the name it's given—schizophrenia, a psychotic episode—those are labels that are put on it. Whether you like it or not you have a psychotic process, and it recurs, and it doesn't have anything to do with your [spiritual] beliefs, or with medications causing it, or with anything else, and that's the reality." He says, "Why are you trying to cut me down and going on like that?" And I say, "I am the voice of reality, that's all I am."

Cathy reports Vern's last incomprehensible behavior to her staff audience, who—momentarily nonplussed—manage only the monosyllabic terms "weird" and "yeah" in response. Staff lament the absence of video equipment, which, in good positivist fashion, they think could "prove" to Vern that his beliefs about "bubbles coming out of his fingers" and a "halo" are false. As Dr. W indicates—authoritatively planting Vern's ineffable experiences on terra firma—staff's job is to use all available means to get Vern to replace his version of his experiences with their psychiatric construction, "psychotic illness."

This clinical task before her, Nadine goes on to discount Vern's claim that people can read his mind. Instead, she nudges him toward the view that he only thinks so, but in reality is reading his own mind. She thus counters Vern's reality by applying an implicit psychoanalytic model that suggests that Vern is essentially interacting with his own repressed fears. His unconscious mind has projected these fears as palpable realities outside himself in sublimated (symbolic) form: he is, in a word, delusional, as is consistent with his psychotic diagnosis.

Vern knows that staff construe his beliefs as indicators of schizophrenic illness, but he will have none of it and accordingly attempts to end this conversation. Still, he apparently decides he has nothing more to lose and nowhere left to hide. Thus he claims he talks to God (which no doubt adds to this clinical picture in Nadine's mind). Further, he seems prepared for the trip back to the hospital, which is the typical psychiatric response to his cosmic voice.

Let us take a brief look at Vern's claim that people are reading his mind: Even if Nadine is right that Vern is only reading his own mind, viewed sociologically (cf. Mead 1934), the individual mind consists mostly of the importation of social processes. So considered, if Vern reads his own mind he must in effect also read others' minds. Further, and this point is probably closest to Vern's meaning, staff's invasive surveillance of the residents' experiences (as documented in Chapter 2) does indeed constitute "reading his mind."

In Chapter 2 Vern claims that these psychiatric practices, especially the drugs, interfere with his spiritual progress. But staff cannot openly grant validity to Vern's cosmic reality and opposition to the psychiatric construction without compromising their status as societal gatekeepers of sanity/insanity. As role models of psychological competence, staff must keep their own private fears (and cosmic realities?) in the closet, and by so doing also safeguard everybody else's taken-for-granted social world. Thus, under Dr. W's directive, Cathy, the self-proclaimed "voice of [psychiatric] reality," hammers Vern's ineffable reality into the box marked psychotic. Her vehemence is proportional to her fear of being outflanked at the border by the Verns of the world. In short, she protests too much. Staff's gay mask of humor slips only to reveal the hard-nosed expression of the border patrol.

On Maureen: Labeled "Borderline"

Dr. W: When working with Maureen, keep in mind one of the problems people like this have is, they over- or undervalue a person. They can quickly idealize somebody as wonderful and great because they've done this magical thing, whatever it happens to be. And other people are bad because they haven't done that thing.

Craig: That's a borderline situation.

Dr. W: Yes it's borderline, and you have to be cautious about what you do.

Craig: She's not interested in investigating anything with us. She's ambiguous about breaking up her relationship, but won't really get into it.

Cathy: She doesn't want to let us in very much at all.

Dr. W: She has borderline features: She tries to split good and bad people. One of the difficulties in working with people like this is a lot seems to work temporarily, and then breaks down.

Cathy: We could at least try to clarify where she's going, what's gonna happen to her son. She just broke up her relationship. We're gonna see a great collapse here.

Craig: We need more historical perspective before this relationship: with her family; did she intend the pregnancy; what was it like for her at school.

Dr. W: She'll resist this. Dr. O pushed her and she got angry. You've got to be real careful. People like her suck you into helping, but won't accept help. They sabotage all attempts to help, dig in their heels, and then blame the helpers.

Dr. W issues a sober warning to the staff: "You have to be cautious about what you do" with "people like this" who "split good and bad people." Dr. W's words show wary respect for Maureen's alleged manipulative power. He almost speaks as a general testing the combat readiness of his troops before facing a wily enemy. Accordingly, staff scramble to get a handle on Maureen, or as Craig puts it, "more historic perspective."

A spector is haunting the psychiatric border—the spector of the "borderline personality." No other label in the psychiatric lexicon elicits so much staff trepidation and vigilance. What is the source of this circumspect fear? The residents so designated are heterogeneous in most respects except for one compelling characteristic: All show a marked ability to find weaknesses in staff personalities and their psychiatric model of reality. Borderlines not only reject some or all of this model, the deficiencies they adeptly expose cast doubt on the expertise of the psychiatric enterprise.

Dr. W correctly points out that labeled borderlines "split good and bad people." Residents like Maureen (the critic of psychiatric models and drugs whom we met in Chapter 2) *do* make sharp distinctions among staff approaches to them. And they make their preferences known to staff in no uncertain terms. In fact, labeled borderlines often take a Ralph Nadar–like consumers' posture toward intervention into their private mental health. They construe psychiatry as a service they pay for, and therefore one over which they ought to have substantial control.

Psychiatric ideology, however, does not allow residents ("patients" or "clients") to have significant influences over the nature of professional services, let alone over the staff who provide them. Rather than influence *over* these practices, the resident is expected to be influenced *by* professional direction. And instead of a consumer role, the resident gets stuck (with a label) to play the "sick role." In essence, doctor knows best. Residents who persistently challenge "father psychiatry" are double trouble. In other words, people who violate rules of public order become "psychotics," and "psychotics" who violate rules of psychiatric order become "borderlines."

Of course, psychiatric authority has always had its opponents among resident populations. And the older psychiatric terms for discrediting such critics were "sociopath" and "character disorder." While sometimes still used interchangeably with the new "borderline" label, the older labels are now more often applied to residents who jockey for narrow personal advantage within the borders of psychiatry, akin to what Goffman called "learning the ropes" (1961:71). The "borderline" designation, however, is usually applied to residents who test the border by occasionally overstepping it. They are clever enough to learn the ambiguities in the rules of the game in order to subvert the game itself.

This "guerrilla warfare" model of borderlines resisting the psychiatric regime may be a limited and exaggerated analogy, since there can be no successful revolutions. But much like a clever child might start an uproar at home by testing his/her parents, a clever so-called borderline promotes discord among staff based on differences in methods of treatment, values, and personalities. Every skilled rebel knows that successful rebellion depends foremost on the ability to exploit the splits in the ruling group, whether parents, government—or psychiatric staff. However, by the same token, ruling groups keep power and lead successful wars by this same strategy of divide and rule.

By so exploiting personal ambiguities and political factions among staff, just a few residents can dampen staff's confidence and decisiveness. They hamper staff's consistency in enforcing rules, and no doubt reduce staff's efficiency in making and implementing policy. Dr. W interprets this loosening of social constraints to mean that borderlines "sabotage all attempts to help, dig in their heels, and then blame the helpers."

Let us examine staff's "attempts to help" in light of their rejection ("sabotage") by labeled borderlines. We begin with (S) Melissa's account, comparing the lives of staff and residents:

> A lot of clients have this emptiness, a lack of love. A big, empty space in their life that I think love has a lot to do with, and friendship, companionship, happiness. Staff have the same thing, but the empty spaces are not quite as big. That makes it a lot easier to deal with. Staff have a lot of the same problems, maybe not to the same degree, but for some reason are able to cope with it better.

Our analysis supports Melissa's point that "staff have a lot of the same problems" as the residents. But missing from her statement is why staff enjoy superior coping ability and do not suffer from these problems "to the same degree." Our analysis suggests this answer: The "empty spaces" in staff lives are "not quite so big" because, just as they did with members of their original families, they vicariously (albeit with altruistic intent) fill them with the pained realities of residents. (S) Lela adds to this concept:

> Sometimes I think there's no difference [between staff and residents] at all. [She laughs.] I think it's a parasitic relationship. As needy as residents are, staff are needy in a reciprocal way. They need to be needed, that's why they're in the profession they're in. A lot of staff are ex-mental patients, or at least a significant number have significant mental health problems. A lot have had heavy problems in the past, but learned more effective coping mechanisms.

The combined accounts of Melissa and Lela explain why labeled borderlines pose a threat to staff: Borderlines are so designated because they reject staff's central self-justifying definition as helpers. This rejection lays bare the helping relationship ostensibly at the heart of psychiatry as in reality a "parasitic relationship," and thus threatens staff "coping mechanisms", which derive from this "need to be needed." Labeled borderlines must implicitly grasp that this compulsive need to help forms the core of staff relationships in their original families and psychiatric work; also, that this need is the source of staff's public sanity and is actualized through staff's parasitic imposition of superior power at their expense.

Staff's often heated and always fearfully circumspect escalation of labeling through the borderline term is then perhaps their ultimate defense against the strongest challenge yet to their legitimacy and sanity. Under siege at the border, the border patrol maneuvers to hold the line. In Chapter 5, we examine some skirmishes.

Notes

1.   This reference is to the book by Richard Bach, *Jonathan Livingston Seagull* (1970), and the film of the same title. It concerns a sensitive and cerebral seagull who departs from his species' typical flight patterns by soaring far beyond their usual vantage point, both physically and spiritually. Humor aside, it is an apt image for Vern.

2.   Walter Benjamin quotes this line from Brecht during his discussion of the latter's political esthetic theory, i.e., "Epic Theater." (Benjamin 1969:265–267).

3.   Charles Manson made this remark during a televised taped interview from prison on NBC in April 1981.

Chapter 5

BORDER DISPUTES

Chapters 3 and 4 examined, among other things, how psychiatric work both exacerbates staff's perceived threat to their sanity and legitimacy and, paradoxically, provides the source, as labeling and dark humor, of their defense. In Chapter 4 we also saw how these defensive strategies escalate when the parasitic relationship underlying the job is exposed—and staff's raison d'être challenged—by the aptly named borderline resident. Here we will focus on face-to-face disputes between staff and residents over the character and location of the border, and explore sources of the descent of battle-weary veteran staff into what is commonly called burnout.

Border Conflict

The following excerpts are from interactions between staff and residents in various work settings, including therapy groups and more informal conversations between (R) Simone and (S) Nigel:

> *Simone:* I don't have to clean up my room if I don't want to. It's my room—so what do you care?
>
> *Nigel:* Other people have to clean up their messes. You agreed to follow the rules. I'm not here to play babysitter. If you can't follow the rules, there's the door.

This conflict typifies the countless minor confrontations between staff and residents that occur daily within psychiatric settings. Simone is living at EPIC in the first place because she has been judged by psychiatric authority as somehow incompetent in following the rules of public order.

Segregated from legitimate society on this basis, Simone is again threatened with social exclusion if she persists in breaking the EPIC house rule requiring that she clean her room.

However, like all of us, Simone requires some stable social environment and affiliation. In accord with this need, as we saw in Chapter 2, most residents come to identify themselves as members of the labeled-psychotic subculture, and the mental hospital of EPIC becomes "home." Simone knows that continued resistance to staff authority could end with second-order ostracism, that is, banishment from EPIC on top of exclusion from legitimate society. Rather than risk this dire outcome, she finally cleans her room as the lesser evil.

Simone faces social censure ostensibly for violating a formal organizational rule mandating clean rooms. The more fundamental rule that governs this situation, however, is the fact that residents must conform to the sick role by following staff directives without resistance. Staff have the power of definition to sanction or banish residents who break this implicit rule, which in fact underlies all aspects of the labeled-psychotic career—from family to psychiatric suite: That is, those people with the official power of definition choose which definitions and rules will prevail, and those people who resist these definitions and rules become the "problem" according to those holding this power.

Disputes between staff and residents often transcend relatively straightforward struggles over particular rules. Rather, they frequently involve more fundamental battles over how best to live one's life, ways of communicating, the nature of social existence, or even the character of the universe itself. We will explore such issues in the following series of conversations between staff and residents. Let us begin by examining firsthand the interaction between (S) Cathy and (R) Vern, about which Cathy reported in Chapter 4:

Cathy: How have you been doing this week?
Vern: [Long pause.] I don't want to talk about it. Could you come back in ten minutes? [Vern is lying in bed and staring out the window with a look of wonderment as though at a palpable presence. His voice is distant and dreamy.]
Cathy: I don't want you to avoid what's going on anymore.
Vern: [Long pause, still staring.] I'm being told not to talk to you.
Cathy: Who's telling you this?
Vern: [Long pause.] I need to see my [Zen] master. [Pause.] Could I go get a cigarette?
Cathy: [Sighs deeply, then speaks in a loud voice rife with frustration,] Look Vern, you can't keep avoiding what's going on with you. It's not some [with irony] "religious breakthrough," it's a psychotic episode. That's

what it's called: psychosis, schizophrenia. You may not want or like it.
I certainly don't like it. But that's what it is. That's the reality.

Vern: [Long pause.] Why are you cutting me down like this?

Cathy heavily confronts Vern for his alleged avoidance of the "reality" of his psychosis. Vern has insisted all along that his experiences are of a religious nature and in no way indicative of mental illness. (Incidentally, Vern readily admits that psychic pain attends his spiritual quest.) No doubt Cathy sincerely believes that her message embodies the reasonable voice of reality against Vern's irrational and stubbornly held psychotic delusions. But Vern experiences her frustrated and angry words, born of weeks of Vern's lack of progress in psychiatric terms, as an assault on his view of reality and his identity, not as a dispassionate evaluation of his condition.

As yet another example of how slippery staff's power of definition over "cosmic" areas can get while under siege, consider the following interaction between (S) Craig and (R) Erin:

Craig: Is there any way you could get a handle on this thing, maybe agree to take your meds without so much fuss?

Erin: People like us believe in God. We can't trust people who give us pills for it. We say "God told us not to go gambling on," and you come up to where, "You better take your meds. We up your medication."

Craig: It's to stop the talking that you're doing to yourself. You look jumbled up, confused. Are you comfortable that way?

Erin: Is it comfortable? Southern Comfortable! Not comfortable, yeah, but I say, "God wants me to do this." God's talking to me and you don't like it—it offends you. I just have to do that.

Craig: I just know when you take your meds you get clearer about things.

Erin: Clearer is queerer! You shouldn't say anything but good. Oh, he says, "God says this," because that's against the law. I'm listening to God, and it always goes so fast that I don't want to push it on anyone because I'm afraid to.

Craig: It's OK to be afraid. Good.

Erin: But when anybody says anything like "God told me to do this," then you just say, "Good," because that's the way you get people to just say that, to cover up their bad deeds down. God has a way of redirecting madness when it comes down to it.

Erin proclaims the existence of a spiritual world where he intimately associates with God. Craig opposes this claim without anger and more subtly than Cathy confronted Vern's similar beliefs when she claimed to be the "voice of reality." Nevertheless, Craig also works to convince Erin that his ideas indicate psychosis and the need for psychiatric drugs to treat it. Erin resists this coercive attempt to reduce his psychic reality to psychotic delusion through his use of the cryptic expression, "Clearer is queerer," and the straightforward, "We can't trust people who give us pills for it" [belief in God]. No wonder he says he is "afraid" to "push" his beliefs on anybody (at once satirizing Craig's imposition of psychiatric dogma). In this psychiatric context such beliefs are indeed "against the law."

Perhaps Erin's claims embody a critique both of psychiatry and the larger societal reality. It is plausible that statements like "God told us not to go gambling on" and "Clearer is queerer" warn us, albeit cryptically, that "comfortable" and "clear" adaptation to the status quo (including everything from nuclear and ecological brinkmanship to world poverty) constitutes "gambling" with our collective planetary fate. Erin constructs psychiatry's essential function as to, in his words, "get people to just say that" [good]. This construct suggests the ideological use of psychiatry to ensure compliance with the status quo both within the psychiatric setting and the larger society. So viewed, psychiatry and society, as Erin puts it, "cover up their bad deeds down." Put within this societal context, the question of who are the more, in Craig's words, "jumbled up" and "confused," staff or labeled residents, becomes yet more problematic. Or, as Erin pointedly concludes, "God has a way of redirecting madness when it comes down to it."

Next, let us examine this more straightforward interchange between (S) Larry and (R) Efrem:

Larry: So you'll be leaving us soon, and you don't have housing yet. Will you go live on the beach?

Efrem: Why not? I've done it before. There's a stream nearby for fresh water and bright starlit skies at night. I have a hugh piece of plastic for protection from the rain, and warm gear for cold nights. It'll be much easier than living in the jungle like I did in [Viet] Nam.

Larry: Is it realistic?

Efrem: Yeah, I think so. I'm not nuts about it, but it's better than that scumbag St. Thomas [cheap hotel]. I'd rather live on the beach.

Larry: You seem defensive about it. Are you blocking exploring your fears around discharge with no place to go?

Efrem: No, I'm not [sarcastic] "blocking my fears" or "defensive." I'm just pissed off. I can't get enough money to buy decent clothes to get a job to get the money to get a house, so I can be respectable like you.

Larry: It sounds to me like you're putting off your fear on all that stuff.

Efrem: I'm not gonna sit here and listen to this bullshit. You're passing judgments on people. I'm not gonna tolerate that. [Efrem then storms from the living area to his room.]

Being practical, Larry reminds Efrem that this discharge from EPIC is imminent and still he has no housing. Efrem (whom we recall from

Chapter 2 as the victim of great personal tragedy while in Viet Nam) responds to this "reminder" with his romanticized plan to live on the beach. It is his poignant attempt to cope with the threat of impending homelessness. Because of the lack of affordable housing in Lakeside, the only viable alternative for ex-EPIC residents often becomes a substandard hotel. While Efrem might be labeled "nuts" by society he is, in his words, "not nuts about" living outdoors, but he clearly prefers this alternative to a "scumbag" hotel.

Efrem boldly claims that his financial rather than his mental condition is the major culprit in his situation. He sees himself as the victim of inherently contradictory social circumstances. As he puts it, "I can't get enough money to buy decent clothes to get a job to get the money to get a house . . . " Larry, however, calls Efrem "defensive" and suggests that Efrem avoids facing his fears by displacing them onto his housing dilemma. He characterizes Efrem's social difficulties as being the result of personal psychological weakness. Faced with Larry's power of definition, Efrem angrily breaks off the interchange by storming from the room.

After the group session is over and Larry has gone, Efrem emerges from his room. (S) Karla asks him to talk with her about the earlier incident with Larry. An excerpt from their conversation follows:

Efrem: That guy's [Larry] a phony elitist asshole.

Karla: Why don't you confront him if you feel that way, instead of exploding and leaving?

Efrem: I don't think he's really with me. He likes to play God like he knows what's going on with everybody. I just didn't want to get into a bigger hassle with him.

Karla: Why couldn't you tell him you are angry because you think he plays God?

Efrem: You can't waste time with guys like him. He's gonna believe he's God come hell or high water.

Karla: Do you make these kinds of assumptions when talking to friends about what they're thinking?

Efrem: No, I don't. I have good communication with my friends, male and female.

Karla: How's this different?

Efrem: You and him don't know me. In this world not everybody's gonna be your friend. How come you're coming on like I'm the bad guy?

Karla: I'm not making you the bad guy. I'm wondering how you can find out what's really going on with Larry. You're making lots of assumptions about him.

Efrem: I can ask him what he's thinking. I have asked him, but I don't think he's honest. I just want him to stay out of my way, and I'll stay out of his. I've been here five weeks. Why are you assuming my assumptions aren't right?

Efrem's characterization of Larry as a "phony elitist asshole" suggests that Efrem sees his conflict with Larry as not amenable to psychological explanation or solution. Rather, he places the dispute in a moral and social context, just as he did the substantive issue of housing from which it arose. Efrem sees Larry as being dishonest regarding his own thoughts and as unwilling to consider another viewpoint. Instead, Larry imposes his psychiatric definitions on Efrem's experiences. In Efrem's words, "I don't think he's really with me. He likes to play God" . . . "passing judgments on people."

Karla answers Efrem's charges by telling him it is better to "confront" Larry with this view of him "instead of exploding and leaving." She then invidiously compares Efrem's hypothetical communication with his friends to his real talk with Larry. Karla hardly takes a dispassionate position on the altercation. On the contrary, by locating the conflict as indicative of Efrem's faulty communication, she ironically joins Larry in imposing a psychiatric definition on Efrem's approach to this situation.

But Efrem is not persuaded. In fact he now includes Karla as part of the oppressive power relation that finds him at the wrong end. As he puts it, "You and him don't know me." While probably willing to grant that staff mean well, Efrem nonetheless sees that staff are neither his friends nor his allies. Instead, the central staff role requiring the reduction of residents' experiences and circumstances to psychiatric categories precludes relations based upon moral equality, a necessary prerequisite in friendship. If Efrem were to confront Larry as if their conflict were a matter between equals, as Karla counsels him to do, this approach would only obscure the reality of unequal power underlying their relationship.

As our analysis has shown, differences of opinion between staff and residents necessarily emerge within this unequal power relation. Thus the former's assumptions are virtually always construed as right and the latter's, as a fait accompli of their labeled status, as wrong. Indeed, Karla implicitly discounts Efrem's claim about Larry's character without fully considering Efrem's experience in the matter, because Efrem has violated the central expectation of the sick role, which is to accept passively staff's power of definition. Thus Efrem is probably right that to approach the conflict with Larry as a psychological dispute between friends will only result in a "bigger hassle" for him through increasing surveillance and darker labeling as "the bad guy." Efrem no doubt knows that his walkout is a futile protest, only adding symptoms to his clinical picture.

Thus we see that the out- and undergunned residents lose their shoot-outs with staff on the border. But the greatest number of challenges to staff authority are less confrontational and more subtly orchestrated. We turn now to explore one such instance between (S) Ken and (R) Keenan:

Ken:	Why do you think I'm using video?
Keenan:	You have lots of toys you want to play with.
Ken:	I can get a whole different idea of what I'm watching without participating.
Keenan:	Watching a lot of depressed people will make me feel better about myself?
Ken:	Is that what you want from this group?
Keenan:	Be a guinea pig for this kind of thing, videotape 'em, do whatever you can.
Ken:	It is like an experiment to sit back and look at it to see what's going on with all these strange folks.
Keenan:	[Disgruntled,] We see ourselves looking gloomy on tape and can say, [ironic] "gee, we ought to be smiling."
Ken:	You can get an objective view of yourself on tape.
Keenan:	This is being reported, huh, what we're trying to be and we're not.
Ken:	It's also a good tool for me. I can see it and figure out what I'm doing.

Keenan answers Ken's question by satirizing the use of video as, in his words, "toys you want to play with." Keenan's comments suggest resistance to the use of this equipment as embodying and deepening the intrusive surveillance documented in Chapter 2. Although he may be "depressed" or "gloomy," Keenan wants no part of being toyed with or used as a "guinea pig" by a staff that he claims does what it pleases. However, Ken discounts Keenan's view of this power relation by never acknowledging, much less exploring, the critical substance of Keenan's position.

Ken responds to Keenan's angry engagement from the position of the detached Olympian observer above and outside the fray: Expressions like "watching without participating" and "an experiment to sit back and look at it" reflect his aloof and evasive position, which implicitly functions to conceal the power relation between staff and residents and so to nullify Keenan's depiction of a clash of interests. Ironically, this (positivistic) method of obscuring underlying power relations is a major way they are reproduced within psychiatric settings.

If this video framework provides a way to arrive at an "objective view" of this situation, as Ken claims, then there are no victors and victims, only equal partners in the disinterested pursuit of truth. Ken's use of the image, "all these strange folks," however, gives away the superior power underlying this spurious claim of neutrality. This blanket labeling of the assembled residents suggests that staff hold and wish to retain their power to define residents as "strange" (psychotic), and so on, with the videotape being one "good tool" for doing so.

Efrem's and Keenan's experiences at the "other" end of the power of definition have taught them much about its anatomy: Even psychiatry's most artfully obscurant devices cannot conceal from them the power relation in which they are the losers. And we have seen that staff's ideological hubris, so easily maintained in private interviews and work settings apart from their charges, becomes much more difficult to sustain in their face-to-face meetings.

It is important to understand, the foregoing critical commentary notwithstanding, that staff intentions for the residents are anything but punitive. My own lengthy work experience (over 8 years) in various psychiatric settings convinces me that sociological criticism of psychiatric work must sensitively address the poignant practical burdens of this tough job. The vast majority of staff are deeply concerned with the welfare of the residents, and very few are authoritarians at heart (as indicated by their outsider identifications in Chapter 3). Quite the contrary, to revisit another point made in Chapter 3, most have altruistic and democratic religious or political values, and are personally inclined to encourage nonconformist actions. Nevertheless, the structural constraints of psychiatric work—including the social–psychological push toward reverse role modeling with its secret threat to staff of their own potential closet insanity—consistently coerce these humanely motivated staff to act in an authoritarian manner.[1] As we have seen, staff learn to defend themselves and society (the border) with their psychiatric ideology, which they believe to be objective. Indeed, only under the guise of objectivity can staff enforce the alleged distinction between their sanity and the insanity of their charges.

But the trials of staff do not end by effectively patrolling the psychic border of themselves, the psychiatric setting, and society. Staff are also required to function as "case managers." With each resident being seen as a "case," staff are expected to pull residents away from their spiritual and other preoccupations and push them toward instrumental goals. As Cathy, in the role of case manager, puts it, "The priority in Vern's life now should be getting a source of income, then housing, food. If he's not interested in getting SSI [disability money from the state], then he can't stay here. The basic thing that we can do for him is get him funded." At the time of this study, the state and county funded treatment of residents at EPIC for a maximum of only six weeks. Given such a short deadline, the frenetic pace required to meet these instrumental goals (quite apart from any attempt at psychic healing) greatly exacerbates the more authoritarian and "mechanistic" aspects of staff relations with the residents—even in staff not so predisposed.

Many staff themselves are extremely critical of this structural aspect of the psychiatric enterprise. For example, Cathy understands that no place exists in our network of social institutions where people are allowed, much less encouraged, to take time out—in the classical sense of "asylum"—from obligations to function in everyday life. To her credit, she is aware that our relentlessly practical culture leaves no room for fully engaging one's spiritual or other impractical concerns, at least not without the attendant stigma of mental illness or otherwise suspect social status.

A few staff, Cathy among them, go so far as to contend that it is psychiatry's central function to engineer people to fit the narrow band of instrumental behavior required for success in the well-oiled everyday world of business as usual. But even these staff critics cannot avoid implementing the psychiatric agenda once they choose the psychiatric worker role over the sick role reserved for the squeaky wheels.

In summary, the psychiatric tools staff employ to control the residents are one and the same as the tools they employ to stay in charge of themselves, namely, psychological vigilance, dark humor, and labeling (except staff use recreational drugs). These strategies enable staff to cope with the growing threat of their own psychological problems (potential closet insanity amplified by reverse role modeling) and job frustration. Staff strategies to safeguard their public psychological competence and social legitimacy at once constitute their work activity, which centrally includes the use of power to ensure the exactly opposite status of the residents. The ironic upshot of these strategies is that staff are unable to achieve the ostensible goal of their work, namely, rehabilitation, which leads to still greater frustration and finally disillusionment. We turn now to explore these processes.

Power Outage

In the following excerpts veteran staff, who have been full-time workers for at least three consecutive years, express their current attitudes toward their work and the residents: we begin with Cathy:

> You get frustrated and depressed in this job. You're exposed to people where you have such an intimate connection, and you don't realize how it works on you. You keep sinking down by seeing all the deprivation, all the underprivilege, all the inability to handle mundane things life tosses you. You start really having difficult stress reactions. It's hard to deal with your own stuff when you put so much into this. If I had a dollar for everyone who really wanted to change, I couldn't eat at MacDonald's today. Not only do we need a few more sick days when we are sick, but we also need "happy days" for when our mood is too good to come to work. We can call up and say, "I'm calling in happy."

Cathy complains that she gets "frustrated," "depressed," and has "difficult stress reactions" from doing her job. She attributes these troubles to her continuous involvement with residents' "deprivation" and "underprivilege." Cathy is aware that her empathetic identification with the intractable circumstances of residents creates a major source of job distress. At this point in her career, however, she is unaware of her complicity in the perpetuation of these circumstances.

When the psychiatric enterprise fails in its mission and everything is up in the air, staff increasingly turn to humor at the expense of the residents, as we saw in "The Joke's on Them" in Chapter 4. Hence Cathy complains that she "couldn't eat at MacDonald's today," because she poignantly perceives that she cannot bet on the residents' willingness or ability to emerge from their plight. And in the burdensome psychiatric roles of "nursemaid" or "case manager," as Cathy puts it, "You keep sinking down."

What is the source of staff's failure to rehabilitate? We have seen that staff's interpersonal strategies, which constitute psychiatric work (e.g., dark humor and labeling), enable them (1) to cope with their own psychic difficulties on the job (feared closet insanity amplified by reverse role modeling) and (2) to meet their compulsive need to be needed as the main motivation for this work (reprising caretaker roles in original families). Obviously, the need to be needed requires reciprocally needy people to avail themselves of this "service." But the price staff must pay for the fringe benefits derived from this parasitic relationship is the ironic subversion of their ability to rehabilitate.

As we outlined earlier in our report of staff's personal unusual experiences outside the work setting, staff's empathetic identification with residents unconsciously includes the latter's labeled status. That is, staff use the same language (e.g., paranoid, schizy, manic, depressive) to describe themselves in a process I call reverse role modeling. Staff's "psychiatrized" identification with the residents' painful circumstances contributes to their failure to alter them. And Cathy's dark humor here just adds to the vicious cycle of negative labels and jokes that ironically create the failure to rehabilitate and resultant sense of futility she bemoans.

Let us examine Cathy's joke about "calling in happy" in light of our analysis. The logic of this joke is that staff's need to work declines in direct proportion to their increasing sense of well-being, which suggests that when staff feel happy they do not need the parasitic source of emotional support that their work provides. In other words, staff use their work as a crutch.

The emotional wear and tear at work leaves many psychiatric workers with diminished resources to, as Cathy suggests, "deal with your own stuff." If her comment is true, it implies why, as seen in Chapter 3, staff frequently indulge in escapist behaviors such as drugs or drinking off the job. If by so doing staff not only forget about the day at work, but avoid their own personal problems, they continue "sinking down" in their private as well as professional lives. But again, in the presence of labeled psychotics, if staff have left unresolved business at home, they can at least believe themselves to be in better shape comparatively. In other words, the parasitic dimensions of psychiatric work that at first attract people to the job become ever more attractive to exploit. Or, if a staff person has a weak leg when s/he starts working in psychiatry, s/he later finds that s/he cannot walk without a crutch, the crutch being the job itself. As Lela confides, "It's amazing to me that people who are supposed to be ordering the divine processes of other people are afraid to look routinely at their own lives."

Let us examine Ken's related observations on his work:

> You can only do this job for a certain time without getting frayed at the edges. There's dissatisfaction from seeing the long-term results here. People get tired. They need to listen to people's problems all the time, and get a distorted view of things. It's a job to come and try to help and assist people, and when that's not working and you don't get paid much, you try to think of other things to blame—the program's administration, etc. Like others who entered the mental health field, I'm disillusioned with the choice. It's frustrating in lots of ways, and people get burned out. It's hard work, and people set themselves up by thinking they [residents] will change more than they do. They won't change because they have a biochemical disorder.

Ken tells us that the day-to-day involvement with psychiatric work erodes initial staff idealism. Here again we notice the futility evident in Cathy's account. In his words, "There's dissatisfaction from seeing the long-term results here. People get tired . . . burned out." Further, he admits that he is "disillusioned with the choice." But what is the source of these poor "long-term results" creating staff futility? Like Cathy, Ken also asserts that staff "set themselves up [for disappointment] by thinking they [residents] will change more than they do." While Cathy blames the failure to rehabilitate on the residents' stubborn resistance to change, Ken's culprit is the intractable nature of the "biochemical disorder" afflicting them. His claim implicitly invokes psychiatry's fundamental paradigm: Psychosis is a (presumably genetic) biological disease of the brain with a biochemical cause and modus operandi. Further, medical science will someday discover its specific etiology and generate a corresponding (biochemical) cure on this basis. In the meantime, Ken offers this balm for staff frustration: Since staff are neither geneticists nor biochemists, they ought not to expect to make much progress in treating this "disorder."

However, our analysis suggests that this psychiatric ideology is able neither to explain nor to cure this painfully stubborn behavior. On the contrary, psychotic behavior is better explained as the ironic effect of this ideology itself. Nevertheless, staff and public alike are indoctrinated to confuse cause and effect here in order (1) to provide an ideological apology for psychiatry's failure to rehabilitate and (2) to keep the power of definition in the "biologistic" hands of the medical and pharmaceutical establishments, which benefit most from this "failure" (really success in light of psychiatry's political mandate to segregate troublesome individuals, thus individualizing and defusing inherently social problems).

The ongoing threat of closet insanity amplified by reverse role modeling becomes increasingly burdensome to staff over time. And, as we have just seen, staff's use of the residents as self-protective props in this ongoing struggle helps to create the additional painful side effect of failure to rehabilitate, which destroys staff's self-identity as helpers. When this recipe for despair is completed, veteran staff's dreams of saving the residents die.

When staff attempts at psychological intervention and rehabilitation ultimately fail, they grasp the bandages endorsed by psychiatry. This medical model legitimizes itself with its biologistic ideology in an increasingly desparate attempt to rationalize why the residents cannot or will not recuperate from their sick role. With such diminishing returns in their frustrated attempts to rehabilitate those unfortunates who will never recross the border, staff descend into what is commonly called burnout. Burnout involves the development of staff's final self-protective coping strategy, which can be usefully thought of as psychological novocaine. We now explore this phenomenon.

Larry and Cathy are talking animatedly about a resident's plan to do volunteer work for the first time. This proposal is a turning point in this resident's motivational picture. They are discussing the resident's strong fears around work issues and ways in which staff might help to mitigate them.

As Larry and Cathy talk, Ken and Nigel, while in close proximity, remain completely outside and nonattentive to the discussion. Instead, Ken is looking out the window with a faraway—even vacant—expression on his face, his eyes fixed in the distance. Similarly, Nigel, staring blankly at the cup of coffee that he cradles in his hands, seems utterly disinterested in the goings on.

Similar scenes reoccur constantly during this research, and incidentally, in every psychiatric facility in which I have worked. Beyond psychological vigilance, dark humor, labeling, and so on, veteran staff assume a stance of detached resignation or indifference as their ultimate defense. Lela sums it up as follows:

> Everybody had a private dream about helping and saving these poor sons of bitches who come here and *could be us* [my emphasis]. At first, people creatively bumped up against the dream, then tangled with it. But none of these dreams got realized, so they gave up.

Lela sees implicitly that burnout is a major defense rife with an unconcern ironically (still) born from failed concern. And she illuminates a major theme in this work: Were it not for the "poor sons of bitches" at EPIC to act as host objects of staff's various defensive and parasitic interpersonal strategies, in Lela's words, the residents "could be us." The border would vanish.

In fact if Ken and Nigel were residents, their withdrawn behavior might be construed as symptomatic of psychosis. Indeed, its remarkable likeness to the blank detachment people tagged "schizophrenic" often display perhaps indicates staff identification with this behavior, or reverse role modeling. In any case, veteran staff often engage in self-protective distancing strategies on a continuum from detached resignation to indifferent withdrawal.

Upon reaching this point some veteran staff bail out of psychiatric work altogether. (The character of the withdrawal strategies replacing the ones documented here requires follow-up research to see if there is "life after psychiatric work.") But most heretofore hands-on "grunts" either aspire to administrative work as the only legitimate structural escape internal to institutional psychiatry, or else they seek the greener pastures of private practice as clinical psychologists, marriage and family counselors, and the like. These noninstitutional psychiatric options offer higher social status, more money, and greater job autonomy. In any case, the vast majority of staff intend someday to leave the discouraging institutional world of "chronic psychosis."

Some staff, however, feel trapped in psychiatric work without other viable options. Over time many have added family responsibilities. Some even achieve fairly respectable remuneration. What begins for many staff as a tentative job while searching for their "real" vocations, for some becomes, often before they know it, their life's work. No doubt like workers in all trades, some staff become prisoners of their psychiatric resumes. It is, after all, what they do. And, though they might protest this judgment through role distance, it is in our culture *who they are*. Kris, a 42 year-old, 15 year veteran, comments: "I got into it out of curiosity and spiritual research. I wanted to see how other people operated. But then it became just more and more a job, and here I am."

There are two basic approaches trapped veterans take to their jobs. Some opt to amplify the defensive strategies already outlined, sometimes including physical abuse of residents (though I am certain this behavior is absent at EPIC), while the overwhelming majority of this group respond as Ken and Nigel do in the above example: they simply tune out the psychiatric environment as much as possible. Interestingly, in accord with our analysis, this may not be altogether bad. Lela documents the effects of this tuning out:

> Clinically, the change has been there's less emphasis on the clinical, and I see that as positive. And the reason there's less emphasis on the clinical is because the clinicians are starting to get burned out. There's less jargon, labels—all that 'treatment planning' crap. I think it goes along with burnout. We just don't have the energy to keep full control. [I ask her if I am correct in understanding her to say that the less energy staff have to do their jobs, the better they do them.] Yes. That's it exactly. [She laughs.] Ironic, huh? When they're burned out, staff treat clients more like people. Or at least since they're tired and avoid them [residents] more, they treat them less like labels.

Lela suggests that burnout causes the psychiatric system to work less efficiently in programming people negatively. *Simply, the more burned out staff become, the less labeling they do.* Our analysis would suggest that "tired" staff who "avoid" residents probably lighten to some extent the intrusive surveillance and probing documented in Chapter 2, thus lending support to Lela's claim. But we learn from psychology that the experience of indifference from significant others is typically felt as rejection or abandonment, not as relief. If burned-out psychiatric workers have managed to keep their light on, unfortunately nobody's home. It is as if, much like the residents, they are sleepwalking through a bad dream in which they must play a role and, so trapped, ironically continue to act out. Roland, a student from the university working at EPIC for the summer, observes:

> Staff are tired, good at heart, loving, busy, trapped. They have much idealism and are good-natured, but because of the way things are, I don't think they are able to express those qualities. They are trapped into being external people by the bureaucracy, their need to give meds. But they have qualities of working with the system. They are all determined to work with it, and have a desire to help. It is not very effective, but admirable.

Roland's terse tour de force remarkably captures what I know as staff's poignant reality. In his terms, these "good at heart, loving, busy" staff with "much idealism" are worn down by "the way things are," the psychiatric "bureaucracy," until "tired" and "trapped," they become "external people." They become hacks of the bureaucracy they are "determined to work with", come hell or high water.

However, this is not the whole story. Amid the darkness, a dogged and authentic "desire to help" keeps saving this bad dream from becoming a worsening nightmare. Yes, they become drones of the system. Yes, they fail. But there are moments of existential beauty. Sometimes, and against all odds, staff even heal the hurt (theirs and the residents'). Here and there "good-natured" and "loving" patches break up the gray institutional horizon. Despite the profound defects extensively documented here, let the record show that moments of this work and these workers—not least the gritty altrusim—shine through as indeed "admirable." I can readily think of worse ways "to do" a life.

But staff typically fail to grasp that it is neither the willful contrariness nor the biological defects of the residents that is the primary villain in this piece. Nor are staff individual villains. They simply know not what they do. Staff's typical blindness to their complicity in the sociological processes documented here is as poignant as it is striking. Cathy, on the cusp of leaving psychiatric work for legal advocacy of labeled psychotics, speaks to this matter:

> They [other staff] believe in the disease model. I used to believe in it. They've got a great heart, are bright, and genuinely care. What they could benefit from is a good sociological education. I don't think they quite get the prominent role they play in stigmatizing. . . . They see themselves as genuinely giving and caring people, and when somebody comes along and says, 'You know, you stigmatize and you damage and you hurt,' they don't really think they do that. They feel that their intentions are pretty pure. It's like trying to convince somebody that they're doing something damaging, when they feel that they're doing the opposite.

This study has tried to meet some of this need for, in Cathy's words, "a good sociological education." Her psychiatric career drawing to a close, Cathy, who confides elsewhere that she is "burned out," now grasps that staff's negatively self-fulfilling ideology ironically creates the very intractable recalcitrance in the residents that staff so decry. Burnout is mainly the result of this central and unsolvable sociological contradiction in psychiatric work: Labeling as the basis of staff's personal and job stability makes their chief work goal—rehabilitation—essentially unrealizable. The central role requirement of psychiatric work unavoidably puts staff in the position of one who puts out the light to curse the darkness. In the final chapter, we review and summarize the key findings in this study.

Notes

1.   This phenomenon calls to mind one of the main points of Zimbardo's (1972) prison experiment at Stanford University: Briefly, the student subjects who were randomly assigned to the roles of inmates and guards took on these role-specific personal characteristics as they played them. That is, guards tended to treat

"inmates" in an authoritarian manner, while inmates became more servile and dependent in relation to the guards. In short, these organizational roles acted as structural sociological constraints that dramatically influenced individual behavior in ways having little or nothing to do with the pre-experiment personalities and self-concepts of the student subjects. The relevance to this study is obvious.

Chapter 6

BORDERLAND

Birds of a Feather

Staff and labeled psychotics alike report that their original families were fraught with psychological and social difficulties, with staff typically adding that they were family caretakers who nonetheless failed to "fix" them. Both groups recount pronounced episodes of refractory sadness, reporting that during such periods ordinary tasks—from domestic chores to work obligations (though career labeled psychotics are rarely employed)—are experienced as an enormous burden. Also, both groups admit to much anxious stress in their everyday lives, with staff locating its sources in the frustrated attempts to rehabilitate their charges for life demands, which they, as role models, also find overly difficult to act out at times. In sum, both staff and their charges show similar patterns of pessimism regarding their personal lives, work, and society in general, as well as fear, futility, stress, felt personal inadequacy, and deep sadness (or in medical psychiatric terms, "depression").

Instructively, staff's problems in handling everyday life abate markedly after entering this work. Before this job, staff report erratic work records not unlike those of the residents. The decision to enter this work, though no doubt (unconsciously) driven by the need to be needed, is typically a default through drift. Rather than a clearly chosen and motivated career option, the role of psychiatric worker often "just happens" to staff—much like the blind descent of the residents into the sick role. And staff who remain so employed do so through lack of alternative technical skills, fear of failure in or distaste for mainstream pursuits, or simply inertia: over the years they have built up a psychiatric job resume that traps them. Further, most staff define themselves as psychologically tenuous and/or look negatively upon dominant cultural realities, toward which they feel marginal.

111

In private talks, staff judgments of the social and psychological short-comings of the residents are also frequently applied to themselves, and are prominently mentioned as empathetic motivators for entering this work. And while staff often express a fear of becoming unable to cope with everyday life, they invariably favorably contrast their painful/unusual experiences with the similar experiences of the residents as putatively sane vs. insane. The residents report no such distinction, however, since the "insanity" of their experiences is a fait accompli of labeled status.

Thus staff are haunted by the spector of loss of status as psychologically competent and socially legitimate persons. Although often muted by humor, staff talk is laced with fearful allusions to prospective personal rejection and failure to reach goals. As crystallized by Lela's comment in Chapter 5 about "these poor sons of bitches who come here and could be us," staff seem to see the psychotic role as but a short step away from their current (quasi–)legitimate status should their interpersonal strategies to safeguard their self-defined marginal legitimacy fail. In short, staff suffer closet insanity.

Closet Insanity

What is closet insanity and how does it emerge in the first place? Staff are required to construct other people's behavior as symptoms of mental illness. The vast majority of staff believe that psychosis is an objective disease entity that causes symptoms in the form of the residents' unusual experiences. Even the minority of staff who resist this model are none-theless threatened by the possibility of its objective truth. Staff fear that if this model is objectively real, then this same model must apply to their own private experiences since, as we saw in Chapter 4, they are often indistinguishable from the public symptoms of the so-called psychotic residents. Thus staff indoctrination into psychiatric ideology (along with reverse role modeling on this basis, which will be summarized below) can create full-blown closet insanity as self-labeling in accord with its prem-ises.

In looking at the sources of this indoctrination, we see that staff are enmeshed daily in an enormous ideological and institutional apparatus, which, of course, they themselves coauthor. The psychiatric enterprise both embodies and has the full weight of governmental, economic, and public legitimacy: The American Psychiatric, Medical, and Psychological Associations, the National Institute of Mental Health, insurance compa-nies and state providers, drug companies, the courts and police agencies, the Family Alliance for the Mentally Ill, and so on, all lend authority to, and thus gain public approval in substantiating, psychiatry's claim to represent social reality.

Thus staff's status and role, not to mention economic survival, are thoroughly integrated within this network of social relations as in fact both their producers and products. Given the total hegemony of psychiatric ideology, it is the rare worker able to resist its sway over his/her thought and practice. The worker who believes him/herself to be unaffected by the psychiatric claim to reality is like a person standing in a hurricane who denies that an ill wind blows.

Is it any wonder, then, that in this atmosphere staff often fear that their own private problems are on the edge of psychosis? As key actors in this "psychiatrization of reality," it could hardly be otherwise. It is as if staff secretly tell themselves in effect, "I don't get crazy or talk crazy in public, so nobody knows that I'm crazy. But everything I've learned about this experience I'm having tells me it's crazy. So maybe I really am crazy." And since staff's daily work reminds them of the bleak consequences that often flow from public displays of unusual experiences, staff hide them in the closet. Unlike people unfamiliar with institutional psychiatry, staff see in the face-to-face example of the labeled residents good reason to fear losing control over their lives. They also glimpse that a crucial difference between themselves and the residents has been their ability (so far) to avoid this contingency. And they take pains to keep it that way.

Reverse Role Modeling

Closet insanity can be fully grasped only in relation to its twin phenomenon, reverse role modeling. All subjective identity is precariously dependent on relations with others. Staff's identity as persons, like that of all people, is importantly rooted in their productive work activity. And if one makes one's living and spends most of one's time in relations constructing and maintaining stigmatized identities, it follows that one's own identity will also show evidence of stigma.

Staff's work activity consists mostly of attributing symptoms of psychosis to the problematic behavior of residents. In time people so labeled come to accept and identify with this construction of their experiences. Eventually, labeled residents in effect say to staff, "So you think I'm crazy, do you? OK, I'll show you something crazy." This cycle ongoingly reinforces "psychotic illness" as "objective reality" for labeled residents.

The problem for staff, however, is that they begin to apply this model to themselves. The chief danger lurks in staff's positivistic assumption that the psychosis ideology that they apply to residents represents objective reality. Staff enter psychiatric work already doubting their psychological competence and social viability. And the labeling of people who publicly manifest painful and odd experiences similar to their own hidden troubles and unusual states leads staff increasingly to hold up the same mirror of insanity to themselves. Staff come to fear that the labeled residents, again in Lela's words, "could be us." Goffman made the point that we can only know the nature of sanity through our knowledge of insanity (1971:366). But it is precisely by knowing, identifying, and identifying with putative insanity—that is, reverse role modeling—that staff cease to be sure of their own sanity. They experience closet insanity.

The only hedge against this conclusion would be significant buffering by everyday people with identities in no way constructed in tandem with the psychiatric apparatus. But such is not the case. With the exception of psychiatrists, staff form a homogenous and ingrown subculture: love, housing, recreational, and other relations are formed almost exclusively with other staff. As we have seen, it is a culturally marginal and "psychoticized" world rife with pessimism, fear, futility, stress, felt inadequacy, and sadness.

However, fear of insanity apropos closet insanity and actual labeled-psychotic status are horses of very different colors. Despite reverse role modeling, insofar as I could tell nobody in my study was labeled psychotic after having become staff. Why is this the case? At least part of the answer is that the personal threat and role strain inherent to staff's subcultural context and work activity also provide, paradoxically, the source of and impetus behind their compensatory strategies to mitigate their distress.

Conclusion

Let me now briefly review the key dimensions of this study: Staff experience closet insanity as exacerbated by reverse role modeling. Closet insanity is staff's private fear and doubt about their psychological competence and social legitimacy. Reverse role modeling is staff's identification with the residents: It results from seeing their own private problematic experience (i.e., closet insanity) mirrored daily in the similar but labeled public behavior of the residents. Since staff believe that the disease model underlying their work is scientifically objective, they apply it (i.e., label) to themselves. Key features of closet insanity and interpersonal strategies to ward it off are:

1. Staff are seriously self-deprecating in private, and prominently use psychiatric terms to refer to their own private experiences, i.e., self-labeling.

2. Staff are hypervigilant toward their own behavior in order to "prove" their sanity relative to the residents, which includes public masking of privately "unusual" experiences.

3. Staff redirect (displace) their felt social psychological inadequacies onto the residents in the following (interwoven) ways:

   a. Derogatory humor in reference to residents.

   b. Serious negative labeling of residents, including prominent use of psychiatric terms.

   c. Pessimism regarding residents' lives and prospects for change, and their own jobs in general (which includes burnout).

   d. Implicit in the other dimensions, staff direct anger toward residents, mostly through subtle but sometimes blatant use of power.

The above strategies typically fail to reduce staff's role strain, and their next step is to distance from direct institutional psychiatric work:

1. Staff move up in the psychiatric hierarchy as administrators, private therapists, and so on.

2. Staff leave psychiatric work altogether.

3. (Rarely) staff enter the labeled-psychotic role.

Finally, in accord with the foregoing analysis, key problematic dimensions of psychiatric work can be summarized:

1. Staff are parasitic vis-à-vis residents as the basis of their (quasi–) legitimate social status and psychological competence.

2. As such, staff are poor role models of competent performance in legitimate society.

Endnote on Critical Ethnography

This work has been motivated by a critical advocacy of people caught in the ever-widening net of institutional psychiatry, including not only how psychiatric ideology and practice constructs labeled psychotics, but also how psychiatric staff are similarly constructed. Although I have presented these dimensions of institutional psychiatry as an integrated picture, particularly in the conclusion, I have tried to avoid serving up "psychiatric reality" on a plate. Rather, I hope I have provided a vivid sketch of psychiatric power relations and the definitional struggles constructing them.

To reiterate a point made in Chapter 1, in my view no person is ever detached or neutral in any social context, but is always engaged, self-awarely or not, in taking a moral and political position—even if only by

default. In this connection, my sociology owes much to the Frankfurt
School and other critical theorists among the various currents of Western
Marxism (see especially Sartre 1968; Held 1982; Warren 1984) in tension
with "postmodernist" influences (see especially Derrida 1976; Clifford
1983; Lyotard 1984). Put baldly, the critical standpoint holds that all
societies to date have been founded upon, and reproduced from, the
class- and patriarchy-based social powerlessness of the vast majority of
people as the dominant feature of everyday life.

During the present late capitalist epoch in the United States and other
advanced industrial societies, this social powerlessness has transcended,
while retaining, its class and patriarchal origins in the form of universal
"commodity fetishism": the tendential reduction of all people and things
to objects of exchange for profit (Marx 1975:71–83). Further, the
"economy" and the "state" (government) have historically fused into an
all-enveloping administrative and technological apparatus (which people
aptly call "the system") organized to promote this universal accumulative
ethic, which increasingly constructs all environmental and cultural contexts in its image, including the most subtle variations in interpersonal
behavior and individual psychic life.

This critical frame of reference, however, can make no warranted
claims to privileged explanatory status. Rather, it must be firmly yet
gently planted in the indigenous cultural and psychological soil of the
ordinary people it allegedly addresses. No doubt its growth will lead to
changes in its perspective, such as the deepening and/or abandonment of
particular aspects of the critique—or even its total transformation into
"something else." In short, critical theory must be grounded ethnograph-
ically. In this connection, I have kept the following (postmodernist)
observations in mind throughout this study:

> There are no integrated cultural worlds or languages. All attempts to posit
> such abstract unities are constructs of monological power. A 'culture' is
> concretely, an open-ended, creative dialogue of subcultures, of insiders and
> outsiders, of diverse factions; a 'language' is the interplay and struggle of
> regional dialects, professional jargons, generic commonplaces, the speech
> of different age groups, individuals, and so forth. . . . [It is] a carnivalesque
> arena of diversity. (Clifford 1983:136–137)

Clifford writes as a kindred spirit of the constructionist standpoint.
However, in my view this "carnivalesque arena of diversity" has always
been shot through with invidiously hierarchical power relations (hardly
"abstract" but actual "monological power") rooted in class and patriarchal
social formations.[1] For me the most telling aspect of Clifford's description
is its allusion to a desirable and achievable future world beyond the
ubiquitous reign of oppressive power in today's carnivalesque market-

place. Nevertheless, we share the basic premises that everybody is responsible for creating and maintaining society (even if coauthored as "masters" and "slaves" and their analogs), and that our social life has no intrinsic meaning apart from our interpretive acts, including, of course, my critical claims. If follows that this book too has no objective meaning apart from our interpretations. The interaction between myself as researcher and writer of this book and the staff and residents of EPIC, and finally, you as its readers, combines to create its meaning and makes all participants coauthors.

But to revisit another point made in Chapter 1, this work, although enabling many native voices to speak to the reader, has not fully embodied coauthorship. While attentive to the intersubjective enactment of social life, my interpretive voice has been authoritative in the "final analysis." The question arises whether raising one's authorial voice in advocacy of others, without always enabling those others to speak for themselves, promotes the goal of democratic self-direction or hinders (or even forecloses) this purpose. It is a crucially important moral and political issue, which critical ethnography must continue to address (Clifford 1983).

In any case, a critical social voice must neither be removed from nor "shout at" ordinary people, which can only lead to its deserved irrelevance by being given a deaf ear. If I am right that the history of human association has always been centrally imbued with forms of domination, then ethnography is inherently critical anyway. No need to shout, for both the potentialities of "what might be" and the present constraints of "what is" are discernible within, for example, my detailed sketch of forms of human association within a psychiatric context. People are enabled to see new possibilities within the present constraints and act to realize them.

What is to be done? Ethnography reminds us that global issues of institutional politics, however mammoth and disturbing, are not just "out there" as "them" or the "system," but are ongoingly and profoundly reproduced "in here" as "us." Institutional circumstances are built up from countless practical face-to-face situations. They therefore can be rearranged in the same way. But with that, we must also soberly realize that all definitions of situations, whether universal or particularistic in scope, emerge within the open-ended and omnidirectional networks of social and material events, including unconscious processes and body sensations. We are unable to grasp in its entirety this complex "fractured totality" within our accounts (Adorno 1983). Inherently lacking omniscient or even privileged awareness of the objective world, we then to a great extent construct ourselves blindly, or as Freud knew, unconsciously and "behind our own backs."

Nevertheless, the quest for meaning is an end in itself, an inherent dimension of our species activity. It is a central paradox of the human condition that, although we cannot fully grasp our rational interests, we are nonetheless predisposed and constrained to try to realize them (Sartre 1956). The practical solution to our dilemma may be to embrace our ambiguity fully: to view the human plenitude as without fixed ideational or material goods, evils, heroes, or villains, either to glorify or to blame. Whatever else freedom can mean, it must include action to explore, affirm, confront, and transform the given reality from as many angles as possible. To our deep bodily minds, "truth" is plural as the endless play of difference.

The key problems of critical ethnography remain:[2] The researcher's ability to get inside indigenous minds is always in doubt, and the totality of any social world is always beyond the author's control and ability to represent fully. As such I encourage you to read against the grain of this and all accounts—to seek out the skirted or buried dimensions in all texts. In the end the meaning of what I have said here depends on your creative activity as readers. And what you do about it depends on your creative action.

Notes

1.   Clifford is sympathetic to this position and addresses it elsewhere (see especially Clifford and Marcus 1986).
2.   The substantive points here closely follow Clifford's (1983) path-breaking examination of ethnographic methods. His orientation has much influenced my approach to this study, and has greatly inspired the methodological direction of my subsequent work.

REFERENCES AND WORKS
OF RELATED INTEREST

Abrams, Richard and Michael Alan Taylor. 1983. "The Genetics of Schizophrenia: A Re-assessment Using Modern Criteria. *American Journal of Psychiatry* 140:171–175.

Adorno, Theodore W. 1950. *The Authoritarian Personality*. New York: Norton.

———. 1974. *Minima Moralia—Refections from Damaged Life*. New York: Seabury.

———. 1976. *The Positivist Dispute in German Sociology*. London: Heinemann.

———. 1982. *Against Epistemology: A Metacritique*. Oxford: Basil Blackwell.

———. 1983. *Negative Dialectics*. New York: Continuum.

American Psychiatric Association. 1987. *Diagnostic and Statistical Manual of Mental Disorders*, 3rd rev. ed. Washington, DC: APA.

Appelbaum, Richard P. 1988. *Karl Marx*. Beverly Hills, CA: Sage.

Archer, Dane. 1984. *Violence and Crime in Cross National Perspective*. New Haven, CT: Yale University Press.

Avineri, Shlomo. 1971. *The Social and Political Thought of Karl Marx*. Cambridge: Cambridge University Press.

Bach, Richard. 1970. *Jonathan Livingston Seagull*. New York: MacMillan.

Barnes, Barry. 1982. *T.S. Kuhn and Social Science*. London: Macmillan.

Barnhart, Edward ed. 1988. *Physician's Desk Reference*. 42nd ed. Oradill, NJ: Medical Economics, Inc.

Bateson, G., D.D. Jackson, et al. 1956. "Towards a Theory of Schizophrenia." *Behavioral Science* 1:251.

Becker, Howard S. 1963. *Outsiders: Studies in the Sociology of Deviance*. New York: Free Press.

———. 1967. "Whose Side Are We On?" *Social Problems* 14:239–247.

Benhabib, Seyla. 1984. "Epistemologies of Postmodernism: A Rejoinder to Jean-Francois Lyotard." *New German Critique* 33:103–26.

Benjamin, Walter. 1969. "Epic Theater." Pp. 265–267 in *Illuminations*, edited by Hannah Arendt. New York: Schocken Books.

Berger, Peter L. 1963. *Invitation to Sociology*. Garden City, NY: Anchor.

Berger, Peter, B. Berger, and H. Kellner. 1974. *The Homeless Mind*. New York: Vintage.

Berger, Peter and T. Luckmann. 1967. *The Social Construction of Reality*. New York, Anchor.

119

Bernstein, Richard. 1976. *The Restructuring of Social and Political Thought.* Oxford: Basil Blackwell.

Bissland, James A. and R. Munger. 1985. "Implications of Changing Attitudes Toward Mental Illness." *Journal of Social Psychology* 125:515–517.

Bleuler, Eugene. 1924. *Textbook of Psychiatry.* New York: Macmillan.

———. 1950. *Dementia Praecox; or the Group of Schizophrenias.* New York: International Press.

Blumer, Herbert. 1969. *Symbolic Interactionism: Perspective and Method.* Englewood Cliffs, NJ: Prentic Hall.

Brandt, Anthony. 1975. *Reality Police: The Experience of Insanity in America.* New York: William Morrow.

Brown, Norman O. 1960. *Life Against Death.* New York: Vintage.

———. 1966. *Love's Body.* New York: Vintage.

Brown, Richard H. 1977. *A Poetic for Sociology: Toward a Logic of Discovery for the Human Sciences.* Cambridge: Cambridge University Press.

Buck-Morss, Susan. 1977. *The Origin of Negative Dialectics: Theodor W. Adorno, Walter Benjamin and the Frankfurt School.* Hassocks, Sussex: Harvester.

Chesler, Phyllis. 1972. *Women and Madness.* New York: Avon Books.

Chu, Franklin D. and S. Trotter. 1974. *The Madness Establishment.* New York: Grossman.

Cicourel, Aaron W. 1964. *Method and Measurement in Sociology.* New York: Free Press.

———. 1970. "Basic and Normative Rules in the Negotiation of Status and Role." In *Recent Sociology,* Volume 2, edited by M.P. Dreitzel. New York: MacMillan.

———. 1974. "Ethnomethodology." In *Cognitive Sociology,* edited by A.V. Cicourel. New York: Free Press.

Clifford, James. 1983. "On Ethnographic Authority." *Representations* vol. 1, no. 2:118–146.

Clifford, James and George E. Marcus, eds. 1986. *Writing Culture: the Poetics and Politics of Ethnography.* Berkeley, CA: University of California Press.

Conrad, Peter and J.W. Schneider. 1980. *Deviance and Medicalization: From Badness to Sickness.* St. Louis, Moseby.

Coulter, Jeff. 1973. *Approaches to Insanity.* London: Martin Robertson. Deleuze, Gilles.

Deleuze, Gilles. 1983. *Nietzsche and Philosophy.* New York: Columbia University Press.

Deleuze, Gilles and F. Guattari. 1977. *Anti-Oedipus: Capitalism and Schizophrenia.* New York: Viking Press.

Denzin, N.K. and S. Spitzer. 1966. "Paths to the Mental Hospital and Staff Predictions of Patient Role Behavior." *Journal of Health and Human Behavior* 7:265–71.

Derrida, Jacques. 1976. *Of Grammatology.* Baltimore: Johns Hopkins University Press.

———. 1979. *Spurs: Nietzche's Styles.* Chicago: University of Chicago Press.

Dilthey, Wilhelm. 1962. In *Pattern and Meaning in History,* edited by H.P. Rickman. New York: Harper and Row.

Doerner, Klaus. 1984. *Madmen and the Bourgeoisie: A Social History of Insanity and Psychiatry.* London: Basil Blackwell.

Dohrenwend, Bruce P. and B.S. Dohrenwend. 1969. *Social Status and Psychological Disorder.* New York: Wiley.

Domhoff, G. William. 1970. *The Higher Circles.* New York: Random House.

―――. 1974. *The Bohemian Grove and Other Retreats.* New York: Harper and Row.

―――. 1983. *Who Rules America Now?* Englewood Cliffs, NJ: Prentice Hall.

Eaton, J. and W. Weil. 1953. "Mental Health Among the Hutterites." *Scientific American* 189:31–37.

Erikson, K. 1962. "Notes on the Sociology of Deviance." *Social Problems* 9:307–314.

Estroff, Sue E. 1981. *Making It Crazy.* Berkeley: University of California Press.

Evans-Pritchard, Edward E. 1937. *Witchcraft, Oracles and Magic Among the Azande.* London: Oxford Unversity Press.

Fabrega, H. 1972. "Concepts of Disease: Logical Features and Social Implications." *Perspectives on Biological Medicine* 15:583–616.

Faris, Robert E.L. and H. Warren Dunham. 1939. *Mental Disorders in Urban Areas.* Chicago: University of Chicago Press.

Feyerabend, Paul K. 1975. *Against Method: Outline of an Anarchistic Theory of Knowledge.* Atlantic Highlands, NJ: Humanities Press.

Foster, Hal, ed. 1983. *The Anti-Esthetic: Essays on Postmodern Culture.* Port Townsend, WA: Bay Press.

―――. 1984. "(Post)Modern Polemics." *New German Critique* 33:67–78.

Foucault, Michel. 1965. *Madness and Civilization.* New York: Vintage.

―――. 1975. *The Birth of the Clinic.* New York: Vintage.

―――. 1979. *Discipline and Punish: The Birth of the Prison.* New York: Random House.

―――. 1980. *Power/Knowledge: Selected Interviews and Other Writings, 1972–1977.* New York: Random House.

―――. 1984. *Foucault Reader: An Introduction to Foucault's Thought.* New York: Random House.

Fraser, Nancy. 1984. "The French Derrideans: Politicizing Deconstruction or Deconstructing Politics." *New German Critique* 33:127–154.

Freeman, Howard E. and O. Simmons. 1963. *The Mental Patient Comes Home.* New York: Wiley.

Freud, Sigmund. 1965. *New Introductory Lectures on Psychoanalysis.* New York: Norton.

―――. 1969. *An Outline of Psychoanalysis.* New York: Harper and Row.

Freund, Julien, 1969. *The Sociology of Max Weber.* New York: Vintage.

Friedson, Eliot. 1970. *The Profession of Medicine.* New York: Dodd Mead.

Fromm, Erich, 1973. *The Anatomy of Human Destructiveness.* New York: Holt, Rinehart and Winston.

Gabel, Joseph. 1975. *False Consciousness: An Essay on Reification.* New York: Harper and Row.

Gallagher, Bernard J., III, 1987. *The Sociology of Mental Illness.* Englewood Cliffs, NJ: Prentice Hall.

Garfinkel, Harold, 1956. "Conditions of Successful Degradation Ceremonies." *American Journal of Sociology* 61:420–424.

————. 1967. *Studies in Ethnomethodology.* Englewood Cliffs, NJ: Prentice Hall.

Geertz, Clifford. 1973. *Interpretation of Cultures.* New York: Basic Books.

————. 1983. *Local Knowledge: Further Essays in Interpretive Anthropology.* New York: Basic Books.

Gibbs, J. 1972. "Issues in Defining Deviant Behavior." Pp. 39–68 in *Theoretical Perspectives on Deviance,* edited by R.A. Scott and J.D. Douglas. New York: Basic Books.

Giddens, Anthony. 1976. *New Rules of Sociological Method.* New York: Basic Books.

Glaser, Barney and A. Strauss. 1967. *The Discovery of Grounded Theory: Strategies for Qualitative Research.* Chicago: Aldine.

Goffman, Erving. 1965. *The Presentation of Self in Everyday Life.* New York: Doubleday Anchor.

————. 1961. *Asylums.* New York: Doubleday Anchor.

————. 1963. *Stigma.* Englewood Cliffs, NJ: Prentice Hall.

————. 1967. *Interaction Ritual.* Chicago: Aldine.

————. 1971. *Relations in Public.* New York: Basic Books.

————. 1974. *Frame Analysis.* New York: Harper and Row.

Goldfrank, Walter L. 1979. *The World System of Capitalism: Past and Present.* Beverly Hills, CA: Sage.

Gove, Walter R. 1982. *Deviance and Mental Illness.* Beverly Hills, CA: Sage.

Gutting, Gary. 1980. *Paradigms and Revolutions: Appraisals and Applications of Thomas Kuhn's Philosophy of Science.* Notre Dame, IN: University of Notre Dame Press.

Habermas, Jurgen. 1972. *Knowledge and Human Interests.* Boston: Beacon.

————. 1973. "A Postscript to Knowledge and Human Interests." *Philosophy of the Social Sciences* 3:XX–XX.

————. 1975. *Legitimation Crisis.* Boston: Beacon.

————. 1981. "Modernity versus Postmodernity." *New German Critique* 22:3–30.

————. 1984. "The French Path to Postmodernity." *New German Critique* 33:79–102.

Haney, Craig A. et al. 1968. "Selective Factors Operating in the Adjudication of Incompetency." *Journal of Health and Social Behavior* 9:233–242.

Held, David. 1982. *Introduction to Critical Theory: Horkheimer to Habermas.* Berkeley, CA: University of California Press.

Hempel, Carl. 1966. *Philosophy of Natural Science.* Englewood Cliffs, NJ: Prentice Hall.

Hochschild, Arlie R. 1983. *The Managed Heart: Commercialization of Human Feeling.* Berkeley, CA: University of California Press.

Hollingshead, August B. and F.C. Redlich. 1958. *Social Class and Mental Illness.* New York: Wiley.

Hughes, Everett C. 1945. "Dilemmas and Contradictions of Status." *American Journal of Sociology* (March): 353–359.

Huyssen, Andreas. 1984. "Mapping the Postmodern." *New German Critique* 33:5–52.

Illich, Ivan. 1976. *Medical Nemesis: the Expropriation of Health.* New York: Pantheon.

Ingleby, David, ed. 1980. *Critical Psychiatry.* New York: Pantheon.

Israel, Joachim. 1971. *Alienation: From Marx to Modern Sociology*. Boston: Allyn and Bacon.

Jacoby, Russell. 1975. *Socail Amnesia: A Critique of Contemporary Psychology*. Boston: Beacon.

Jameson, Fredric. 1972. *Marxism and Form: Twentieth Century Dialectical Theories of Literature*. Princeton, NJ: Princeton University Press.

———. 1981. *The Political Unconscious*. Ithaca, NY: Cornell University Press.

———. 1984. "The Politics of Theory: Ideological Positions in the Postmodernism Debate." *New German Critique*. 33:53–65.

Jay, Martin. 1973. *The Dialectical Imagination: A History of the Frankfurt School and the Institute of Social Research, 1923–1950*. Boston: Little, Brown.

Kiesler, Charles A. and Amy E. Sibulkin. 1987. *Mental Hospitalization: Myths and Facts about a National Crisis*. Newbury Park, CA: Sage.

Kitsuse, John I. 1962. "Societal Reaction to Deviant Behavior: Problems of Theory and Method." *Social Problems* 9:247–56.

Kohn, M.L. and J.A. Clausen. 1955. "Social Isolation and Schizophrenia." *American Sociological Review* 20(3):265–273.

Kolakowski, Leszek. 1968. *The Alienation of Reason: A History of Positivist Thought*. New York: Doubleday.

Kornhauser, Arthur W., ed. 1965. *Mental Health and the Industrial Worker—A Detroit Study*. New York: Wiley.

Kovel, Joel. 1980. "The American Mental Health Industry." Pp 72–101 in *Critical Psychiatry*, edited by D. Ingleby. New York: Pantheon.

Kraepelin, Emil. 1904. *Lectures on Clinical Psychiatry*. London: Baillorie, Tindall, and Cox.

Kuhn, Thomas S. 1970. *The Structure of Scientific Revolutions*. Chicago: University of Chicago Press.

Laing, Ronald D. 1967. *The Politics of Experience*. New York: Pantheon.

———. 1985. *Wisdom, Madness and Folly*. New York: McGraw-Hill.

Laing, R.D. and A. Esterson. 1970. *Sanity, Madness and the Family*. New York: Penguin.

Lemert, Edwin M. 1962. "Paranoia and the Dynamics of Exclusion." *Sociometry* 25:2–20.

———. 1967. *Human Deviance, Social Problems and Social Control*. Englewood Cliffs, NJ: Prentice Hall.

Lyotard, Jean-Francois. 1984. *The Postmodern Condition: A Report on Knowledge*. Minneapolis: University of Minnesota Press.

Manning, Peter K. and M. Zucker. 1976. *The Sociology of Mental Health and Illness*. Indianapolis: Bobbs-Merrill.

Marcuse, Herbert. 1966. *Eros and Civilization*. New York: Vintage.

———. 1968. *One-Dimensional Man*. Boston: Beacon.

———. 1969. *Reason and Revolution*. Boston: Beacon.

Marx, Karl. 1975. *Capital*, Volume 1. New York: International Publishers.

Matza, David. 1969. *Becoming Deviant*. Englewood Cliffs, NJ: Prentice Hall.

McHugh, Peter. 1970. *Defining the Situation: The Organization of Meaning in Social Interaction*. New York: Bobbs-Merrill.

Mead, George H. 1934. *Mind, Self, and Other*. Chicago: University of Chicago Press.

——. 1938. *The Philosophy of the Act*. Chicago: University of Chicago Press.

Mehan, Hugh and H. Wood. 1975. *The Reality of Ethnomethodology*. New York: Wiley.

——. 1976. "De-secting Ethnomethodology." *The American Sociologist* 11:13–21.

Nagel, Ernest. 1961. *The Structure of Science*. New York: Harcourt, Brace and World.

Nehamas, Alexander. 1985. *Nietzsche: Life as Literature*. Cambridge, MA: Harvard University Press.

Niedradzik, Krystyna and R. Cochrane. 1985. "Public Attitudes Towards Mental Illness—The Effects of Behavior, Roles, and Psychiatric Labels." *International Journal of Social Psychiatry* 31:23–33.

Nietzsche, Friedrich. 1967. *On the Genealogy of Morals. Ecce Homo*, edited by Walter Kaufmann, New York: Vintage.

Nunally, James. 1961. "What the Mass Media Present." In *Popular Conceptions of Mental Health*, edited by J. Nunally. New York: McGraw Hill.

O'Connor, James. 1987. *The Meaning of Crisis*. New York: Basil Blackwell.

O'Kane, John. 1984. "Marxism, Deconstruction and Ideology: Notes Toward an Articulation." *New German Critique* 33:219–247.

O'Neill, John. 1972. *Sociology as a Skin Trade: Essays Toward a Reflexive Sociology*. London: Heinemann.

Orwell, George. 1954. *Animal Farm*. New York: Harcourt, Brace and World.

Parsons, Talcott. 1951. *The Social System*. New York: Free Press.

——. 1975. "The Sick Role and the Role of the Physician Reconsidered." *Health Society* 53:257–278.

Phillips, Derek. 1963. "Rejection: A Possible Consequence of Seeking Help for Mental Disorders."*American Sociological Review* 28:963–972.

Plunkett, R.J. and J.E. Gordon. 1960. *Epidemiology and Mental Illness*. New York: Basic Books.

Polanyi, Karl. 1944. *The Great Transformation*. Boston: Beacon.

Pollner, Melvin. 1987. *Mundane Reason: Reality in Everyday Sociological Discourse*. Cambridge: Cambridge University Press.

Radnitsky, Gerhard. 1970. *Contemporary Schools of Metascience*. Chicago: Henry Regnery.

Reich, Wilhelm. 1970. *The Mass Psychology of Fascism*. New York: Farrar, Straus and Giroux.

Robinson, Paul A., ed. 1969. "Herbert Marcuse." Pp. 147–244 in *The Freudian Left*, edited by Paul A. Robinson. New York: Harper and Row.

Rose, Gillian. 1978. *The Melancholy Science: An Introduction to the Thought of Theodor W. Adorno*. London: MacMillan.

Rosenhan, D.L. 1973. "On Being Sane in Insane Places." *Science* 179(19):250–258.

Rosenthal, Robert. 1966. *Experimenter Effects in Behavioral Research*. New York: Appleton-Century-Crofts.

Rosenthal, Robert and L. Jacobson. 1968. *Pygmalion in the Classroom*. New York: Holt, Rinehart and Winston.

Roth, Martin and J. Kroll. 1986. *The Reality of Mental Illness.* Cambridge, England: Cambridge University Press.

Rothman, David. 1971. *The Discovery of the Asylum.* Boston: Little, Brown.

Rubin, Lillian. 1976. *Worlds of Pain.* New York: Basic Books.

Ryan, Michael. 1982. *Marxism and Deconstruction.* Baltimore: Johns Hopkins University Press.

Sagan, Carl. 1985. *Cosmos.* New York: Ballantine Books.

Sampson, H., S.L. Messinger, and R.D. Towne. 1961. "Schizophrenia and the Marital Family: Identification Crises." *Journal of Nervous and Mental Diseases* 133:423–29.

———. 1962. "Family Processes and Becoming a Mental Patient." *American Journal of Sociology* 68:88–96.

Sarbin, Theodore and J.C. Mancuso. 1980. *Schizophrenia—Medical Diagnosis or Moral Verdict?* New York: Pergamon.

Sartre, Jean-Paul. 1956. *Being and Nothingness.* New York: Philosophical Library.

———. 1968. *Search for a Method.* New York: Vintage.

———. 1969. *The Critique of Dialectical Reason.* New York: Vintage.

Scheff, Thomas J., Ed. 1975. *Labeling Madness.* Englewood Cliffs, NJ: Prentice Hall.

———. 1984. *Being Mentally Ill: A Sociological Theory,* 2nd ed. New York: Aldine.

Schneider, Joseph W. and J.I. Kitsuse. 1984. *Studies in the Sociology of Social Problems.* Norwood, NJ: Ablex.

Schneider, Michael. 1975. *Neurosis and Civilization: A Marxist/Freudian Synthesis* New York: Seabury.

Schutz, Alfred and T. Luckmann. 1973. *The Structures of the Life-world,* Volume 1. Evanston, IL: Northwestern University Press.

Scull, Andrew T. 1977. *Decarceration: Community Treatment and the Deviant—A Radical View.* Englewood Cliffs, NJ: Prentice Hall.

———. 1981. *Madhouses, Mad-doctors, and Madmen.* Philadelphia: University of Pennsylvania Press.

———. 1983. *Social Control and the State.* Philadelphia: University of Pennsylvania.

Sennett, Richard and J. Cobb. 1973. *The Hidden Injuries of Class.* New York: Vintage.

Shershow, John C. 1978. *Schizophrenia.* Cambridge, MA: Harvard University Press.

Shroyer, Trent. 1975. *The Critique of Domination.* Boston: Beacon.

Simmel, Georg. 1955. *Conflict* (translated by K.H. Wolf). New York: Free Press.

Spector, Malcolm and J.I. Kitsuse. 1987. *Constructing Social Problems.* Hawthorne, NY: Aldine de Gruyter.

Spitzer, Stephan P. and N.K. Denzin. 1968. *The Mental Patient: Studies in the Sociology of Deviance,* vol. 2.

Srole, Leo et al. 1962. *Mental Health In the Metropolis. The Midtown Manhattan Study,* Volume I. New York: McGraw Hill.

Staten, Henry. 1984. *Wittgenstein and Derrida.* Lincoln: University of Nebraska Press.

Sullivan, Harry S. 1953. *The Interpersonal Theory of Psychiatry.* New York: Norton.

Szasz, Thomas S. 1961. *The Myth of Mental Illness.* New York: Harper and Row.

———. 1970. *The Ideology and Insanity.* New York: Doubleday Anchor.

———. 1976. *Schizophrenia: The Sacred Symbol of Psychiatry.* New York: Basic Books.

———. 1984. *The Therapeutic State.* Buffalo: Prometheus.

Taber, M. et al. 1969. "Disease Ideology and Mental Health Research." *Social Problems* 16:349–357.

Temerlin, M.K. 1968. "Suggestion Effects in Psychiatric Diagnosis." *Journal of Nervous and Mental Disease* 147:349–53.

Terkel, Studs. 1975. *Working.* New York: Avon.

Thio, Alex. 1988. *Deviant Behavior.* New York: Harper and Row.

Thomas, W.I. 1931. "The Relation of Research to the Social Process." In *Essays on Research in the Social Sciences.* Washington, D.C.: Brookings Institution.

Thompson, E.P. 1967. "Time, Work-discipline and Industrial Capitalism." *Past and Present* 38:56–93.

Torrey, E. Fuller. 1974. *The Death of Psychiatry.* Radnor, PA: Chilton.

Vandenburgh, Henry W. 1979. "Critical Theory and Mental Health and Illness." Unpublished graduate student paper in Sociology, University of California, Santa Cruz, California.

Wagner, Roy. 1981. *The Invention of Culture.* Chicago: University of Chicago Press.

Waitzkin, H. and B. Waterman. 1974. *The Exploitation of Illness in a Capitalist Society.* Indianapolis: Bobbs-Merrill.

Wallerstein, Emmanuel. 1978. *The Capitalist World Economy.* Cambridge: Cambridge University Press.

Warren, C.A.B. and J.M. Johnson. 1970. "A Critique of Labeling Theory from the Phenomenological Perspective." In *Theoretical Perspectives on Deviance,* edited by R.A. Scott and J.D. Douglas. New York: Basic Books.

Warren, Scott. 1984. *The Emergence of Dialectical Theory.* Chicago: University of Chicago Press.

Watson, G. Llewellyn. 1982. *Social Theory and Critical Understanding.* Washington, D.C.: University Press of America.

Weber, Max. 1958. *The Protestant Ethnic and the Spirit of Capitalism.* New York: Scribner.

———. 1966. *The Theory of Social and Economic Organization.* New York: Free Press.

Wellford, C. 1975. "Labeling Theory and Criminology: An Assessment." *Social Problems* 22:332–345.

Wilde, W. 1968. "Decision-making in a Psychiatric Screening Agency." *Journal of Health and Social Behavior* 9:215–21.

Wittgenstein, Ludwig. 1953. *Philosophical Investigations.* New York: MacMillan.

———. 1974. *On Certainty.* New York: Harper and Row.

Yarrow, M.R. et al. 1955. "The Psychological Meaning of Illness in the Family." *Journal of Social Issues* 11(4):12–24.

Zimbardo, Philip G. et al. 1972. "The Pathology of Imprisonment." *Society* 9:6.

Index

Borderlines, labeled, 90–93
Burnout, 107–109

Capitalism, 7, 116
Closet insanity of staff (*See also*
    Interpersonal strategies)
  burden of, 106
  comparison of, with residents'
    insanity, 71–76
  disclaimers against, 76–77
  emergence of, 112–113
  experiences of, 56–59
  psychic pain in, 71–74
  reverse role modeling and, 113–114
Community psychiatry, 9–11
Comparative analysis, of staff and
    residents, 71–76
Conflict
  Efrem (R) vs. Karla (S), 99–100
  Efrem (R) vs. Larry (S), 98–99, 100
  Erin (R) vs. Craig (S), 97–98
  Keenan (R) vs. Ken (S), 100–102
  Simone (R) vs. Nigel (S), 95–96
  Vern (R) vs. Cathy (S), 96–97
Constructionist theory
  positivism and, 8
  social problems and, 3–5
  social reality and, 2
Coping, 60–61 (*See also* Interpersonal
    strategies)
Critical ethnography, 115–118
Critical theory
  description of, 5
  social problems and, 5–6
  sociology and, 116

Dark humor (*See* Humor)
"Demential praecox," 8
Detached resignation, 106–107
Diagnostic interviews
  with residents
    Efrem, 27–30
    Janice, 26–27
    Terry, 23–25
  with staff
    Dr. Williams, 66–69
    Melissa, 18–19
Drugs, psychiatric, 33–35

Eastside Psychiatric Intervention
    Center (*See* EPIC)
Emotional pain (*See* Psychic pain)
EPIC (Eastside Psychiatric
    Intervention Center) *See also*
    Residents; Staff)
  fictional name and location of, 11
  organizational roles of staff at,
    13–14
  research at
    codes used in, 17
    dimensions of, 14–15
    empirical questions in, 17
    ethnography and, 115–118
    field methods of, 15–19
    observer effects of, 19–20
  setting of
    organizational, 11–13
    physical, 14–15
Escapism, 104–105
Ethnography, 115–118

127